Keto Diet Cookbook for Women After 50

The Definitive Nutritional Guide to Lose Weight Quickly with The Best, Tastiest, And Easy to Make Low-Carb Recipes, That Will Increase Your Self-Esteem

Amy Newton

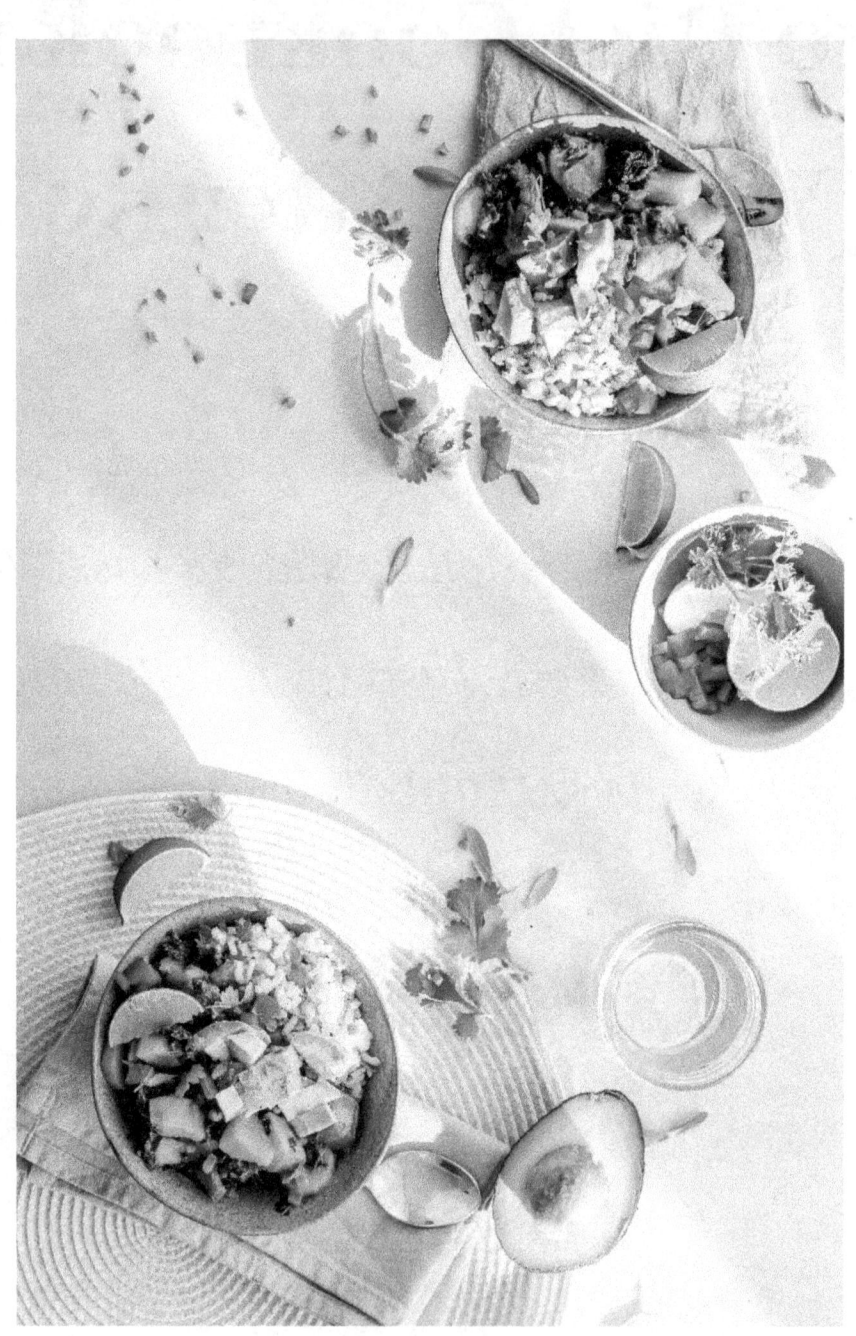

© Copyright 2020 by Amy Newton - All rights reserved.

The following Book is reproduced below with the goal of providing information that is as accurate and reliable as possible. Regardless, purchasing this Book can be seen as consent to the fact that both the publisher and the author of this book are in no way experts on the topics discussed within and that any recommendations or suggestions that are made herein are for entertainment purposes only. Professionals should be consulted as needed prior to undertaking any of the action endorsed herein.

This declaration is deemed fair and valid by both the American Bar Association and the Committee of Publishers Association and is legally binding throughout the United States.

Furthermore, the transmission, duplication, or reproduction of any of the following work including specific information will be considered an illegal act irrespective of if it is done electronically or in print. This extends to creating a secondary or tertiary copy of the work or a recorded copy and is only allowed with the express written consent from the Publisher. All additional right reserved.

The information in the following pages is broadly considered a truthful and accurate account of facts and as such, any inattention, use, or misuse of the information in question by the reader will render any resulting actions solely under their purview. There are no scenarios in which the publisher or the original author of this work can be in any fashion deemed liable for any hardship or damages that may befall them after undertaking information described herein.

Additionally, the information in the following pages is intended only for informational purposes and should thus be thought of as universal. As befitting its nature, it is presented without assurance regarding its prolonged validity or interim quality. Trademarks that are mentioned are done without written consent and can in no way be considered an endorsement from the trademark holder.

Table of Contents

- **INTRODUCTION** 5
- **CHAPTER 1.   WHY THE KETOGENIC DIET?** 9
  - What Is Ketosis? 9
  - Is the Keto Diet Healthy for People Over 50? 10
  - Getting into Ketosis 11
  - The Ketogenic Lifestyles 21
  - How to Know You Are in Ketosis 28
- **CHAPTER 2.   WHY THE KETO DIET FOR WOMEN AFTER 50?** 29
  - Body Changes After 50 30
  - Benefits of Ketogenic Diet for Seniors 31
  - Ketogenic Diet and Menopause 33
  - Most Common Mistakes and How to Fix Them 36
- **CHAPTER 3.   INTERMITTENT FASTING AND KETO DIET** 38
  - What Is Intermittent Fasting? 38
  - Intermittent Fasting on the Keto Diet 40
  - Intermittent Fasting for Seniors 42
- **CHAPTER 4.   KETO RECIPES** 49
  - Breakfast Recipes 49
  - Lunch Recipes 68
  - Dinner Recipes 88
  - Poultry Recipes 113
  - Side Dishes & Snacks 134
  - Salads Recipes 151
  - Soup Recipes 165
  - Smoothies Recipes 181
  - Desserts Recipes 190
  - Condiments And Sauces Recipes 202
- **CHAPTER 5.   THE 21-DAY MEAL PLAN** 214
- **CHAPTER 6.   FORBIDDEN FOOD LIST** 218
  - Starch and Carbs 218
- **CHAPTER 7.   KETO SHOPPING LIST FOR SENIORS** 224
  - Keto Ingredients 224
  - Aging and Nutritional Needs 225
- **CONCLUSION** 230

Introduction

Did you ever want more energy in your day and feel better and look better? Many people have come up with a simple diet to achieve a better life. Sounds unrealistic, I know. However, it is conceivable to acquire energy, feel better, and look better and change your eating habits. There's no magic pill. Rather it's as simple as developing an eating plan that gives the nutrients your body needs.

What's that magic plan of eating? It is called the Ketogenic Diet. This eating method is not so new and has existed for thousands of years. Modern society, unfortunately, selects convenience foods that are generally loaded with carbohydrates and refined sugars.

Eating is often done on the go today. Convenience is what sells, and the producers satisfy the demands of the consumers. These convenience foods come with preservatives, artificial coloring, added refined sugar, salt, and processed grains. Though our schedule may be convenient, these foods are not convenient for our bodies to process.

The ketogenic diet may sound complicated and technical; however, very literally, this diet feeds your body foods that can be processed more easily. The human body is made to function using fuel food, which, in effect, gives us energy. The ketogenic diet optimizes that process.

A ton of readers may not think about the ketogenic diet. In the broadest terms, a ketogenic diet is an eating pattern that makes the liver produce ketone bodies, moving the body's digestion away from glucose and towards fat use.

In particular, a ketogenic diet limits sugar under a specific level (normally 100 grams for each day) and instigates a progression of alterations. Protein and fat intake differ, as indicated by the calorie counter's objective.

Be that as it may, a definitive determinant of whether an eating regimen is ketogenic is the nearness (or absence) of starches. The body runs under 'ordinary' dietary conditions on a blend of starches, protein, and fat. When starches are expelled from the eating regimen, the little stores in the body quickly become exhausted.

The ketone bodies are a result of the fragmented liver corruption of FFA. They fill in as fat-inferred, non-starch fuel for tissues, such as the cerebrum. When ketone bodies are shaped at quick levels, they aggregate in the circulation system, which triggers the creation of a metabolic state called **ketosis**. Simultaneously, the utilization and creation of glucose diminish. The breakdown of protein to be utilized for vitality alluded to as 'protein saving' is diminishing. With an end goal to lessen the fat-to-muscle ratio while staying away from loss of fit weight, numerous people are pulled in to eat less.

The alterations referenced above are activated primarily by ketogenic diets, affecting two hormones: insulin and glucagon. Insulin is a storage hormone that moves supplements out of the circulation system into target tissues. For instance, insulin puts away glucose as glycogen in the muscle, and FFA puts away triglycerides in the fat tissue.

Glucagon is a fuel-preparing hormone that invigorates the body to separate the put-away glycogen to give glucose to the body, especially in the liver. As the eating regimen takes out starches, insulin levels lessening, and glucagon levels rise. This causes an expanded arrival of FFA from fat cells and expanded consuming of FFA in the liver.

What inevitably adds to the advancement of ketone bodies and the keto-metabolic state is the fast consuming of FFA in the liver. Some different hormones are likewise influenced, notwithstanding insulin and glucagon, all of which assist utility of fat over sugars.

The body has four fuel sources: carbohydrates, fat, protein, and ketones. But what exactly are ketones? **Ketones** develop as fat is broken down inside the body. The effect of a ketogenic diet is that fat and ketones are the body's principal source of power. Consuming more fats, moderate protein, and minimal carbohydrates are the secret to following a ketogenic diet. In this way, the body can be in a state of nutritional ketosis.

You need to explore the benefits/risks with your doctor before you start any diets. It's essential to consider the effect a diet can have on your body and your health. This will help you pick a safe diet and deliver optimum results. Eating a ketogenic diet is not simply eating a diet low in carbohydrates. Consider not counting carbohydrates but being aware of your body and responding to the foods you eat. Do you just give yourself the nutrients you need?

A ketogenic diet is a lifestyle change and a change of mindset. The blood sugar levels can drop rapidly when the body uses carbohydrates to convert glucose to energy. The signs are sugar and starch hunger and cravings.

Drops in blood sugar are minimized on a ketogenic diet. This is because fats and ketones are used as fuel rather than as quick carbohydrates to burn. Foods that cause cravings for sugar, salt, and fats hinder weight loss. These addictive foods trigger food over-consumption which never give a true sense of satisfaction. Most often, the culprits are processed foods.

These foods can be avoided on a ketogenic diet, and so are the resulting cravings and hunger for junk food. Instead of calorie counting, adhere to foods that are found in nature and are easy to pronounce. Inflammation is caused by foods such as grains, dairy, and refined sugar. Inflammation hinders weight loss and causes your body to build up toxins. The toxins will be removed after the ketogenic diet starts, and inflammation will decrease.

In this book, you'll be exposed to some of the most easily prepared mouth-watering recipes, and before you know it, the ketogenic diet will cease to be a diet; it will become a way of life.

As you will find, a ketogenic regimen is about high fat, low sugars, and a sound measure of protein, permitting your body to depend on fats for energy instead of consuming the starches. Also, the additional time you spend on the program, you'll feel progressively solid.

However, the important thing is when you begin the ketogenic diet. It's the consistency that is something to remember. Of course, when the opportunity presents itself, you can find it difficult not to indulge in the occasional cheat meal, for instance during the holidays or on an outing with friends. While your body should be able to bounce back fully once you return to the diet, you must adhere to it as strictly as possible to sustain a high metabolic rate.

Chapter 1. Why the Ketogenic Diet?

What Is Ketosis?

Ketosis is a metabolic process in which the body uses fat as energy instead of carbohydrates. Additionally, ketosis is also a state in which mild amounts of ketones are present. The keyword here is mild. In sharp contrast to this, ketoacidosis is a complication of unmanaged type 1 diabetes and it is a dangerous, potentially fatal condition.

According to *Healthline*, ketoacidosis is a "condition resulting from dangerously high levels of ketones and blood sugar." This surplus in ketones—around ten times the amount of when the body is in ketosis—results in the blood becoming abnormally acidic and this, in turn, affects organ function.

In a nutshell, ketoacidosis is a dangerous complication of a disease when your bloodstream gets flooded with immense amounts of ketones. In contrast, ketosis is a healthy metabolic state caused by a low-carb diet like the keto diet.

The Keto Diet Is Dangerous

Speaking of danger, many seem to dismiss the ketogenic diet as a dangerous fad. In reality, the ketogenic diet is not inherently dangerous and as long as you're careful, there's absolutely nothing to be concerned about.

Be careful to avoid unwanted dangers by gradually easing into the diet, ensuring you stay hydrated, and hitting your daily macros. It does have downsides, but many beneficial things contain potential downsides. It's just a matter of actually understanding how it works and being cautious. Avoid rushing into it blindly, hoping that it is a magic weight loss formula. As with any diet, you should always be aware of its effects on your body, and consult your physician if you are concerned.

The Keto Diet Is The Best Way To Lose Weight

With all the hype surrounding the keto diet, you can be forgiven for thinking it is the best way to lose weight. You may even think it is the only way to lose weight, sort of like the be-all, end-all of diets. Well, it definitely isn't the panacea of weight-loss diets because it's different for everybody. In fact, a 2015 study published in the journal *Cell* posted that the blood sugar responses to the same foods vary among people so there is no diet that's perfect for everybody. Having said all that, the best diet is still the one you can consistently stick with.

The keto diet has been shown to be very effective for losing weight and it offers a lot of health benefits. Still, not everybody can benefit from keto, and misconceptions about it are common. Above all, it's always best to consult a doctor before trying out new diets.

Is the Keto Diet Healthy for People Over 50?

If you are a woman over the age of 50, you may be much more involved in weight loss than you were at the age of 30.

Several women undergo a decelerating metabolism at a pace of about fifty calories a day. It may be exceedingly difficult to regulate weight gain by increasing the metabolism when combined with less activity, muscle deterioration, and the propensity for intensified cravings.

To help lose weight, there are several diet choices available, but the ketogenic diet has been among the most common lately. With the aim of making the body burn its own fat resources more effectively, a ketogenic diet is a diet that involves reducing carbohydrates and increaseing fats. Analysis has demonstrated that keto diets are good for general health and weight reduction. Keto diets have facilitated certain individuals to lose excess body fat without extreme desires that are characteristic of most diets. Any patients with type 2 diabetes have already been shown to be able to use keto diets to manage their symptoms. At the core of the keto diet are ketones.

As an alternative energy source, the body creates ketones, a fuel compound, while the body is low on blood sugar. Ketones are created when you lower the carb consumption and eat just the correct amount of protein. Your liver will convert body fat into ketones as you consume keto-friendly foods, which are then used by your body as an energy supply. You are in ketosis as the body utilizes fat for energy supply. In certain situations, this causes the body to significantly raise fat burning, which helps to eliminate pockets of unnecessary fat. This fat-burning approach not only lets you shed weight, but it can also fend off cravings during the day and eliminate sugar crashes.

Getting into Ketosis

Please note that the steps outlined below are formulated with the general public in mind. If you have a pre-existing condition, then it's better for you to consult a healthcare provider before attempting the ketogenic diet.

Step 1 – Determine Your Big WHY

Determining your big WHY is the first step in any diet regimen – not just for the keto diet. Ask yourself why would you choose to deviate from your normal, and perhaps more satisfying diet? What do you want to achieve?

A person who wishes to change his or her diet typically wants to achieve one of the four goals:

- Lose weight
- Gain weight or build muscle
- Improve overall health
- Improve performance (for athletes)

You may be choosing the keto diet for the same reason as the majority: you want to lose weight. The good news is, not only will it help you to achieve this goal, but it can also bring about an improvement in overall health as well as an improved physical performance.

However, that said, if you want to build muscle, keto may not be the best option for you. This is because initially, carbohydrates have a huge role when it comes to muscle recovery. That's not to say you can't see results with keto, though. It's just that it may not seem the way to begin with. Once you have determined your big WHY, hold on to that thought as you progress along the diet's rocky road. As you may have already heard, the Ketogenic diet is NOT easy. A lot of people wind up giving up in the middle simply because it's too hard for them to follow the restriction in carbohydrates and the kinds of fats allowed.

As most inspirational speakers say, 'when you're about to give up, think about why you started.' So, take some time to deliberate about your goal, as it's really important.

Step 2 – Determine Your Total Caloric Goal

The next step after finding your goal is to calculate how many calories you need daily. The number of calories you need is definitely determined by your goal. For the purposes of this book, we're going to assume that you'd like to lose weight.

So how do you compute your caloric requirement if you want to lose weight? We'll cover that in this section, but first, we need to discuss the calories themselves.

What Are Calories?

One definition of calories is this: it is the amount of energy needed to raise the temperature of 1 kg of water by 1 degree Celsius. That's quite complicated, right? So, we'll settle for this definition: calories are energy. Without calories, we would not be able to survive.

Since calories are energy, we need to "burn" them to get energized. Think about climbing a mountain without proper sustenance. Do you think you'd have enough energy to reach the summit? Probably not if you didn't have enough calories to burn in the first place.

Calories are so crucial to our lives, that our body chooses to store them within muscle and fat tissues. If we eat food and we didn't use the calories in that food, then our body will store them for future use. Where will our bodies store them? Most likely in those 'cushiony' places like the tummy, breast, buttocks, thighs, and even arms. Yup – unused calories or those calories that we didn't burn are stored as the unwanted fats or – the preferred option- the wanted muscles for those who want to beef-up.

It's a little morbid, but try imagining a person who has stopped eating for a really, really long time. You would probably see him as someone who's still alive but is all 'skin and bones.' Well, that is so because since he wasn't eating, the body naturally took his calorie reserves from his muscles and fats. It's the body's own way of making sure that you survive in case some circumstances prevent our intake of food.

Calories and Losing Weight

Now that we've cleared up the role of calories in survival, it'll be easier for us to understand their role in losing weight. In the ketogenic diet or in any other diet regimen, you need to work your calories in order to maintain, gain, or lose weight.

Simply put, if you want to maintain weight, then you need to take in as many calories as you burn. If you want to gain weight, then you need to take in more calories than you burn. And finally, if you want to lose weight, you need to burn more calories than you take in.

Let's say that again: if you want to lose weight, then you need to burn more calories than you take in. That's the simplest formula, and it applies even in the ketogenic diet.

Now, we've arrived at the most-awaited part: how do we compute the number of calories that we need?

Computing Your Total Caloric Goal

Before we teach you how to find your total caloric goal, we need to emphasize something – there's no one-size-fits-all formula for this. Your friend's caloric requirement is different from yours because you have different activities.

To compute your caloric goal, we need to take into consideration your activities because that's how we're going to find out how many calories you burn in a day. The term for the number of calories we burn in a day is **total daily energy expenditure** or simply, TDEE.

Now, TDEE is broken down into several components, namely BMR, TEF, NEAT, and TEA. We will discuss all except for TEF since you won't be able to use it to compute for the TDEE. TEF stands for the Thermic Effect of Food or the calories we burn after digesting food.

Basal Metabolic Rate (BMR)

The **basal metabolic rate** is the number of calories needed for the activities within our body. You see, you just don't need calories for when you move, bike, or hike. You also need calories for your heart to beat, for your lungs to perform gas exchange, or for your body to regulate temperature.

In other words, BMR is the number of calories you need outside the calories you require to move.

Non-Exercise Activity Thermogenesis (NEAT)

NEAT is the number of calories you need if you want to make little movements, such as fidgeting, blinking, and moving your fingers.

Thermogenic Effect of Activity (TEA)

TEA is the number of calories you need for more physically-taxing activities, such as running, jogging, or swimming.

Now, to compute your TDEE or the total amount of calories you need to consume in a day, you must multiply your BMR with your Activity Factor (AF). Here's a table for your AF:

Activity Level	Description	AF
Sedentary	Little to no exercise at all	1.1
Light	Light exercise 1 to 3 times weekly	1.2
Moderate	Moderate exercise 2 or more days weekly	1.35
Very Active	Hard exercise 3 or more days weekly	1.4
Extreme	Exercising twice a day or more	1.6

As for calculating your BMR, it's going to be a tedious process, so you can head over online for faster results.

Sample Computation:

Let's have an imaginary person who wants to lose weight as an example. Let's call her Jenny. Jenny has the following AF and BMR:

$$AF = 1.35$$

$$BMR = 1,451 \text{ calories}$$

Again, to get her TDEE (Total Daily Energy Expenditure), you need to multiply her AF with her BMR. In this example, her BMR is already provided. The computation goes like:

$$\text{TDEE} = 1.35 \times 1{,}451 \text{ calories}$$

$$\textbf{TDEE} = \textbf{1{,}958.55 calories}$$

Take note that TDEE is her required caloric intake in a day – it's not her supposed caloric intake if she wants to lose weight. If Jenny would like to lose weight, then she needs to consume less than her TDEE.

Caloric Intake if you want to Lose Weight

Remember that if you want to lose weight, you need to consume fewer calories than your TDEE! But don't go around not eating because that's going to cost you a lot. Experts say cutting down your TDEE by 15 or 20 percent is a good starting point. We call this the "lessening of TDEE" as a calorie deficit.

If you want a sustainable weight loss or a weight loss that you can follow through in the long run, then cut down your TDEE by 15% for at least 3 weeks and see how it goes. Simply use this formula:

$$\text{TDEE} \times 0.85$$

In Jenny's case, you can compute:

$$1{,}958.55 \times 0.85 = \underline{\textbf{1{,}665.02}}$$

This means that for Jenny to lose weight, she needs to take 1,665.02 calories instead of her TDEE which is 1,958.55. She'd like to try this caloric goal for a period of 3 weeks to see if it's working or not. If it's working, she may go on with the same calorie level, or if she wants to see more results, she may cut down more of her calories (from 15%, she may now reduce it by 20%)

But the most crucial thing here is you must choose a calorie deficit that you are comfortable with. If you don't feel well when cutting your intake by 15%, try to cut it down by 10%. What's important is you're starting somewhere.

Step 3 – Incorporate Your Caloric Goal into the Ketogenic Diet

Phew! That was such a lengthy discussion, but hopefully, you got something good from it. To recap: remember that our first step is to identify your overall goal, and the second is to calculate your caloric goal.

The third step involves incorporating that caloric goal into the ketogenic diet. And to do that, you need to think about your macros, or the sources of your calories; namely carbohydrates, fats, and proteins.

You see, your macros give different amounts of calories. Refer to the table below:

Macros	Calories
1 gram of carbohydrates	4
1 gram of proteins	4
1 gram of fats	9

Now, you need to identify which macros you need for a keto diet. What we mean is you have to decide where most of your calories will be coming from. Given that it's keto, you'll need to heavily rely on fat; hence a ratio that looks like this is a good starting point:

60 – 75% calories must come from fat

15 – 30% calories must come from protein

5 – 10% calories must come from carbohydrates

So, let's go back to our previous example of Jenny. Say Jenny wanted to start the keto diet and she wants to ease her way into to. This means she doesn't want anything drastic, like getting 75% of her calories from fat, 20% from protein, and 5% from carbs. She feels that too few carbs will make her extremely weak and sick.

Again, she wants to ease slowly into the diet regimen. So, Jenny decides to go for these macros:

60% of her calories will come from fats

30% of her calories will come from proteins; and

10% of her calories will come from carbohydrates

Now remember, her caloric goal is dictated by her goal to lose weight. It was **1,665.02**. That means:

60% of 1,665.02 calories will come from fats

30% of 1,665.02 calories will come from proteins; and

10% of 1,665.02 calories will come from carbohydrates

The result would look like this:

999 calories will come from fats

500 calories will come from proteins; and

167 calories will come from carbohydrates

The only thing left to do now is to convert these figures into grams. You can use the table of Macros and Calories above. Simply divide 999, 500, and 167 by 9, 4, and 4 respectively. Here's the computation:

Fats: 999 calories / 9 calories = 111 grams of fats

Proteins: 500 calories / 4 calories = 125 grams of proteins

Carbohydrates: 167 calories / 4 calories = 41.75 grams of carbs

IMPORTANT: This computation only serves as an example. Some computations on the internet make use of your Body Mass Index and that could be even more accurate. Some even ask you to choose how many carbs you'd like to eat in a day, although many experts say that limiting it to 35 grams daily is okay! If in doubt, consult a doctor or a dietician.

Step 4 – Prepare Your Keto Checklist and Meal Plans

Since you have already established your goals, it's now time to prepare your keto food checklist and meal plan. To do this, you'll need to know what foods are allowed on Keto and what foods aren't.

Step 5 – Prepare for Keto Flu

Once you have started the ketogenic diet, remember that some changes in your body will happen. Don't be surprised!

Think about it: you are shifting from taking most of your calories from carbs to cutting carbs back to as little as 35 grams a day! In the first few weeks, you might feel really sick because of keto.

This sickness is often called the keto flu because of a variety of flu-like symptoms you experience as your body transitions from carb-burning to fat-burning. The symptoms include:

- Insomnia
- Sugar cravings
- Sore muscles

- Dizziness
- Confusion
- Irritability
- Nausea
- Cramping
- Stomach aches

Don't worry though. There are ways to feel better when you develop the keto flu. You can:

- Increase your water intake, and add a pinch of unrefined salt to one or two of those glasses of water.
- Increase the sodium, potassium, and magnesium levels in your diet.
- Turn to MCT (medium-chain triglyceride) oil for more energy
- Go for a morning walk or other low-intensity exercise
- Get enough sleep
- Reduce stress through meditation

Finally, if you experience the keto flu, do NOT perform strenuous exercises and do not consume too much protein. You can also try to prevent the keto flu by gradually reducing your carb intake before you fully embrace the ketogenic diet. What this means is before officially starting on keto, you can try reducing your carb intake until you reach your actual keto computations for fats, proteins, and carbs.

Key Takeaways

To start keto:

Step 1 – Identify your goal or reason for going keto.

Step 2 – Calculate your caloric goal; you can refer to the suggested website for easier computation.

Step 3 – Incorporate your caloric goal into the macros of the ketogenic diet. You can refer to the recommended websites for easier calculations.

Step 4 – Prepare your keto checklist and meal plans

Step 5 – Prepare for keto flu

Remember that there's no one-size-fits-all formula for keto. You need to consider YOURSELF when thinking about starting this diet regimen.

The Ketogenic Lifestyles

There are keto diet laws that will help you meet your targets for weight reduction. A high-fat and very-low-carb eating plan, the ketogenic diet, may be challenging to initiate. It's definitely a dramatic deviation from the way you live today. After all, the traditional American daily diet is heavy in sugars and refined foods. Yet there are a number of people following the keto diet that places the body in a condition of ketosis. That's what occurs when the carb-burning state in the body flips to a fat-burning one, a move that can induce weight loss and has also been credited with the regulation of type 2 diabetes. The key rules that beginners should bear in mind before beginning the keto diet are provided below:

Rule #1: Must Have Knowledge of Foods to Eat and Avoid

You'll severely restrict carbohydrates by implementing a keto meal schedule. Starting off the day with between 20 and 30 grams of carbohydrates.

Be sure you know what foods mainly include sugars, fat, and protein, so you can make the best decisions. It's not all pizza, spaghetti, popcorn, sweets, sweets, and ice cream, including carbohydrates, for instance. Beans can have protein, but they are strong in carbohydrates as well. Carbs are often present in berries and vegetables. Meat (protein) and pure fats such as butter and oils (including olive oil and coconut oil) are the other items that do not include carbohydrates.

Rule#2: Carefully Think About Your Relationship with Fat

People fear fat because they've been told it's going to kill them. On the usage of fat, there are several contrasting opinions. It gets confusing to know how precisely to consume then. It would also be good to recognize that food is more than a single ingredient, and it is the general consistency of the diet that matters. Start making minor changes to what you consume every day, such as buying a sandwich on lettuce leaves and subbing green vegetables for fries, to plan for a high-fat diet, which may feel difficult at first. Then go for a non-starchy vegetable instead of potatoes or rice for your dinner. With more oil, such as olive or avocado oil, start cooking. Realize the old dieting patterns just don't make sense on a keto diet, so you won't get enough fat, such as having a basic skinless grilled chicken breast.

The plurality of nutritionists accepts that more monounsaturated fats, present in plant-based foods such as avocados and olive oil, should be consumed since they are known to be partially responsible for the heart-healthy benefits of the Mediterranean diet.

You should also substitute foods such as chips once a day for a handful of almonds, use avocados to produce smooth cookies and sauces, and liberally use olive oil to sauté vegetables and create salad dressings. Start moving out carbs slowly to bring in the fat.

Rule#3: Change Your Views of Protein

Most of the keto diet's more popular myths are that you should consume as much protein as you'd like. But this is not a diet where you just aim at carbohydrates. You will need to maintain the consumption of moderate protein. It is important to turn protein into glucose, so overeating protein will bring the body out of ketosis. Think of the amounts, rather than the other way around, as a tiny piece of meat covered by a large quantity of fat.

Rule#4: Improve Your Cooking Skills

Since too many things are off-limits, keto causes you to consume more frequently at home. That's a positive thing since you just don't know how many restaurants use oil or sugar. However, when you feed at home, you have a lot of influence on what goes into your meals. You ought to inform yourself of numerous keto-approved recipes, and selecting four to five recipes for ingredients that you know you'll enjoy is strongly recommended. You won't wait around asking whether to feed this direction and then switch to carbohydrates.

The keto diet is more about growing your calorie consumption, and most of us consume so many refined foods abundant in fat anyway. A diet like this helps you to take out those items that can further decrease your excess weight and boost your nutrition.

While most big sources of carbohydrates are taken out by keto, you can take out refined carbs while also eating nutritious whole grains such as brown rice and oats.

Only make sure to pay attention to the portions. Five to six 1-oz portions of whole grains a day are suggested (for example, one serving is one slice of whole-wheat bread). For pasta and rice dishes, incorporate vegetables like spaghetti squash and zucchini.

Rule#5: Bulletproof Coffee Is A Remarkable Keto Drink

It is created in your coffee by mixing coconut oil and butter. This drink will help hold your appetite at bay, leaving your flexibility to prepare your next meal.

Just remember that coconut oil has the ability to raise LDL, or "poor" cholesterol levels, so you'll certainly want to avoid this drink whether you have heart problems or are at an elevated risk for it because of family or personal health background.

Rule#6: Learn About Side Effects-The Keto Flu and Use Fermented Foods

There's one major side effect you ought to be prepared for—the keto flu—given all the attributes of a ketogenic diet (like weight loss). Keto flu applies to the time when the body is reacting to burning fat for energy when you start the diet. There are certain persons who have no trouble with it, and some are depressed. Your limbs may feel severely lethargic in the first week or 10 days. Maybe going upstairs sounds hard. Maybe you're struggling with emotional fog. Also, because of a shift in fiber consumption, keto induces constipation or even diarrhea. For that reason, when your week is not wild with commitments and responsibilities, you can choose a start date; select a slower period when you can relax as required. In the same lines, within the first week or two, you'll want to be careful to take things easy with exercise when your body needs longer to change between fuel sources to consume fat rather than carbohydrates.

Cutting out vital fiber sources, such as whole grains and fruits, will make you feel pretty backed up, so it's not a surprise that a popular keto symptom is constipation.

That's when fermented vegetables come in to help. Good bacteria in your stomach keep things good and serve like a probiotic. Try kimchi, sauerkraut, or pickles to bring something to your diet. Kefir and yogurt are both excellent probiotic alternatives, but they're not usually fermented.

Rule#7: Maintain A Suitable Level of Electrolytes to Prevent Keto Side Effects

Your kidneys excrete more water and electrolytes during ketosis. Be sure that you get the sodium and potassium that your body requires to operate properly. Salt the food, drink salted bone broth, and consume asparagus, kale, bell peppers, and arugula for non-starchy vegetables.

Rule#8: Increase Your Intake of Non-Starchy Vegetables

Nutritionists say that keto gets us to consume more non-starchy vegetables, such as broccoli, asparagus, and spinach because most adults don't get enough vegetables.

These vegetables help the digestive system provide the fiber it craves. And while most vegetables fill you up with fewer calories, there are also lower BMIs among people who consume vegetables daily.

Basically, you can't always overdo things on the vegetables, as long as nutritionists are concerned, just strive to provide at least one cup for any meal.

Rule#9: Intermittent Fasting

In certain keto circles, intermittent fasting is all the rage. It might sound drastic, but throughout the day, the most common therapies typically allow you to eat food for eight hours. Your body gradually burns off all the carb reserves (i.e., glucose and glycogen) during fasting cycles and continues to consume body fat for energy.

Rule#10: Accept When Keto Might Not Be Right for You

Now that ketogenic diets have become common, several keto hybrid diets, including variations focused on plants, have appeared. One is the ketotarian diet which is primarily plant-based, but contains eggs, ghee, and fish and shellfish choices. You should be mindful about it since, on a ketogenic diet, you should not consume beans or lentils, and because of their carbohydrate content, nuts and seeds are also limited. Therefore, you're only just left with some tofu, and you're going to have to focus on low-carb protein powder. There are also medical problems that may make you think twice before beginning keto. Before attempting it, at least speak to the doctor. These involve persons on insulin, as well as those on elevated blood sugar or high blood pressure oral and noninsulin injectable drugs. Also, dealing with GI difficulties may be an obstacle in the beginning. Constipation is one of the side effects of a ketogenic diet, but if that's a problem, there's a serious excuse not to be on this very low-fiber diet. Finally, a ketogenic diet may be too restrictive for you if current personal dietary limitations enable you to eliminate foods such as wheat, poultry, nuts, grains, or seafood. In an otherwise stringent diet, coming from a position of removal will make a diet extremely challenging to obey.

Rule#11: Inform Your Family About Your Weight Loss Targets

Your strategy should be to inform them. During family dinners, you will not be willing to consume what they're consuming, so you'll want to brace them (and yourself) for what your new routine may look like. As this diet is mostly only carried out in the short term (three to six months), you should tell them that it is temporary.

If people understand the expectations of a keto diet, it does not harm, because they are less inclined to force workplace snacks or to propose sharing a side of fries while you're out for dinner.

Rule#12: Need to Have A Post-Keto Plan

A keto diet is not a diet that can last long. It's designed to be short-term. A couple of days each year, some individuals go on a keto diet; some may do it to shed weight and improve their dietary patterns. Your overall aim should be to shift your food to a healthy trend that requires consuming lesser wheat, pasta, rice, and sugar as well as more non-starchy vegetables.

When the keto diet is done, think of what it would be like for you. Why can this temporary diet be used as a springboard to boost your long-term health?

Rule#13: A Fatty Breakfast

They go about their day attempting to adopt the plan. Then they hit the evening and remember they didn't get sufficient fat and have to drink thick cream to cover for it, whereas most people struggle at keto. Instead, what you can do is fill as much of the fat as possible at breakfast. Typically, that's coffee or black tea with 1 tablespoon of butter, MCT oil, or ghee in it. You can have mushroom coffee with some of those fats in it if you want to change things up a little, and you may even check MCT oil powder if you have catastrophe pants with the usual oil. But if you want to have daily breakfast, it's still pretty easy: bacon, avocado, eggs, and maybe a couple of keto coffees.

That's 15 grams of fat if you have three eggs. Four pieces of bacon are around 15 grams or so. Another 15 grams is half of an avocado. Each keto coffee cup is 14 grams. First thing in the morning, the target is to have at least one-third of the fat for the day, because you don't have to think about it any later. You should measure the TDEE and work out the amount and then find out what 70 percent of it is in grams of fat. If your weight is 160 pounds and you want to reduce to 150lbs, you can have 150 g of fat all day long, and you can aim for at least 50 g for breakfast. If your weight is 110 and you aim to hit 100, you can have 100 grams of fat for the day and at least 33 grams for the breakfast shoot.

While most of the breakfast items we've seen are in the 15-gram range of fat, we may make the regulation easier: split your target weight by 30, round it up, and that's how many "carb parts" you can get for breakfast.

A fat serving is:

4 slices of bacon

3 eggs

Half of an avocado

One tea or coffee with 1 tbsp of butter/MCT oil/ghee/heavy cream

Right now, this sounds like a lot of thought, but until you work out what your number is and look for a breakfast mix which you prefer, you don't have to worry again about it. Now, I'm looking forward to creamy, buttery java, and you're definitely going to notice that you love the flavor, too.

Rule#14: One Fat Per Meal

From your fatty meats and fatty breakfast, you can get much of your calories, but you always need to combine a little more to the meal to ensure you reach your target.

Adding cheese, salad sauce, or nuts is the best method to do this. You'll get the fat you like if you can have a handful of cheese, a handful of pecans or walnuts, or add 1 to 2 teaspoons of olive oil and ranch dressing to your meal.

Bottom Line

The easiest approach is to have a measuring kit for blood ketones. This helps you to see very plainly whether you're in ketosis or not. Moreover, you know how good you adhere to your eating.

What if one of these experiments is used and it looks that the diet doesn't work? Are you just not gaining weight, or are you not losing weight in keto? Three points must be attempted in order:

Making sure you really don't eat carbohydrates

No sweeteners, no sauces or carb dressings, no high-carb nuts.

Reduce the consumption of meat

Maybe you have so much meat, so cut it down to one and a half fist.

Lower the average consumption

You don't want to decrease the fat amount, but the last option to do (mainly if you don't lose weight) is to just eat none of it all. Meet these instructions, and you should have no trouble slipping into ketosis and remaining there. The first week can be a bit tough, but you'll notice it's a pretty simple diet to survive on after that.

How to Know You Are in Ketosis

To understand whether you are in ketosis, you can take tests of urine or blood which will display a higher level of ketones in the body. But then, rather than depending on these tests, you can get a whole picture when you observe the following symptoms. They are:

- Increased thirst and urination along with dry mouth – When the diet changes to a low-carbohydrate one, it can cause water retention in the body. In a diet with a high amount of carbohydrates, the extra carbs are stored as glycogen in the liver. Glycogen is bound to water molecules.

  So, when you shift to a low-carb diet, the amount of glycogen stored gets diminished, which in turn means you are storing less water and therefore a higher chance of dehydration. So, there is a loss of excess fluid when you move to a high-fat diet and thus can make you feel thirstier. There would be increased urination also since electrolytes are also flushed out since the ketogenic diet is naturally diuretic.

- Keto breath – Since ketone bodies called acetones escape through our breath, there is a possibility of making a person's breath smell fruity. The smell disappears in the long run. The ketone bodies can also escape through sweat.

Chapter 2. Why the Keto Diet for Women After 50?

The health benefits of this diet are not different for men or women, but the speed at which goals are reached does differ. As mentioned, women's bodies are a lot different when it comes to the ways they can burn fats and lose weight. For example, by design women have at least 10% more body fat than men. It doesn't matter how fit you are; this is just an aspect of being a woman that you must consider. Don't be hard on yourself if you notice that it seems like men can lose weight easier — that's because they can! What women have in additional body fat, men typically have in muscle mass. This is why men tend to see faster external results because that added muscle mass means that their metabolism rates are higher. That increased metabolism means that fat and energy get burned faster. When you are on keto, though, the internal change is happening right away.

Your metabolism is unique, but it is also going to be slower than a man's metabolism by nature. Since muscle is able to burn more calories than fat, the weight just seems to fall off of men, giving them the ability to reach the opportunity for muscle growth quickly. This should not be something that holds you back from starting your keto journey. As long as you are keeping realistic bodily factors in mind, you won't be left wondering why it is taking you a little bit longer to start losing weight.

Another unique condition that a woman can experience but a man cannot be Polycystic Ovary Syndrome (PCOS), a hormonal imbalance that causes the development of cysts. These cysts can cause pain, interfere with normal reproductive function, and, in extreme and dangerous cases, burst. PCOS is actually very common among women, affecting up to 10% of the entire female population. Surprisingly, most women are not even aware that they have this condition. Around 70% of women have PCOS that is undiagnosed. This condition can cause a significant hormonal imbalance, therefore affecting your metabolism. It can also inevitably lead to weight gain, making it even harder to see results while following diet plans. In order to stay on top of your health, you must make sure that you are going to the gynecologist regularly.

Menopause is another reality that must be faced by women, especially as we age. The majority of women begin the process of menopause in their mid-40s. Men do not go through menopause, so they are spared from yet another condition that causes slower metabolism and weight gain. When you start menopause, it is easy to gain weight and lose muscle. Most women, once menopause begins, lose muscle at a much faster rate, and conversely, gain weight despite dieting and exercise regimens. Keto can, therefore, be the right diet plan for you. Regardless of what your body is doing naturally by way of processes like menopause, your internal systems are still going to be making the switch from running on carbs to deriving energy from fats.

Because the keto diet reduces the amount of sugar you are consuming, it naturally lowers the amount of insulin in your bloodstream. This can actually have amazing effects on any existing PCOS and fertility issues, as well as menopausal symptoms and conditions like pre-diabetes and type 2 diabetes. Once your body adjusts to the keto diet, you are overcoming the things that are naturally in place, preventing you from losing weight and getting healthy. Even if you placed your body on a strict diet, if it isn't getting rid of sugars properly, you likely aren't going to see the same results that you will when you try going keto. This is a big reason why keto diets can be so beneficial for women.

As we've deliberated, carbs and sugar can have a huge impact on your hormonal balance. You might not even realize that your hormones are not in the balance until you experience a lifestyle that limits carbs and eliminates sugars. Keto is going to reset this balance for you, keeping your hormones at healthy levels. As a result of this, you'll find that you will feel better, healthier, and younger, by implementing the simple steps that will tune your body into processing excess fats for energy. You'll build muscle, lose fat, and feel much more energy to get through your days.

Body Changes After 50

Many people attribute aging to sickness and pains, but this assumption doesn't have to be. Getting old doesn't mean a decline in good health. Although when you begin to age, it comes with some levels of decline in the systematic function of the body. This decline in bodily functions doesn't have to be painful and isolating.

The sad reality is that many seniors don't have the proper diet guide to help balance their body and keep it functioning optimally at old age. Furthermore, many seniors without a proper diet often engage in the consumption of high carb diets which is neither healthy nor helpful for people of age 50 and above.

With a proper keto diet plan, old age isn't as unfortunate as many see it. A good diet plan will help your physical and mental health as you age.

Benefits of Ketogenic Diet for Seniors

For aging women, menopause will bring severe changes and challenges, but the ketogenic diet can help you switch gears effortlessly to continue enjoying a healthy and happy life. Menopause can upset hormonal levels in women, which consequently affects brainpower and cognitive abilities. Furthermore, due to less production of estrogen and progesterone, your sex drive declines, and you suffer from sleep issues and mood problems. Let's have a look at how a ketogenic diet will help solve these menopausal side effects.

Enhanced Cognitive Functions

Usually, the hormone estrogen ensures the continuous flow of glucose into your brain. But after menopause, estrogen levels begin to drop dramatically, and so does the amount of glucose reach the brain. As a result, your functional brainpower will start to deteriorate. However, by following the keto diet, for women over 50 the problem of glucose intake is circumvented. This results in enhanced cognitive functions and brain activity.

Hormonal Balance

Usually, women face major symptoms of menopause due to hormonal imbalances. The keto diet for women over 50 works by stabilizing these imbalances in hormones such as estrogen. This aids in experiencing fewer and bearable menopausal symptoms like hot flashes. The keto diet also balances blood sugar levels and insulin and helps in controlling insulin sensitivity.

Intensified Sex Drive

The keto diet causes a surge in the absorption of vitamin D, which is essential for enhancing sex drive. Vitamin D ensures stable levels of testosterone and other sex hormones that could become unstable due to low levels of testosterone.

Better Sleep

Glucose disturbs your blood sugar levels dramatically, which in turn leads to poor quality of sleep. Along with other menopausal symptoms, good sleep becomes a huge problem as you age. The keto diet for women over 50 not only balances blood glucose levels, but also stabilizes other hormones like cortisol, melatonin, and serotonin, warranting improved and better sleep.

Reduces Inflammation

Menopause can upsurge the inflammation levels by letting potential harmful invaders in our system, which result in uncomfortable and painful symptoms. Keto diet for women over 50 uses the healthy anti-inflammatory fats to reduce inflammation and lower pain in your joints and bones.

Fuel Your Brain

Are you aware that your brain is composed of 60% fat or more? This infers that it needs a larger amount of fat to keep it functioning optimally. In other words, the ketones from the keto diet serve as the energy source that fuels your brain cells.

Nutrient Deficiencies

Aging women tend to have higher deficiencies in essential nutrients such as iron which leads to brain fog and fatigue; Vitamin B12 deficiency which leads to neurological conditions like dementia; fat deficiency that can lead to problems in cognition, skin, and vision; and Vitamin D deficiency that not only causes cognitive impairment in older adults and increases the risk of heart disease but also contributes to the risk of developing cancer. On a keto diet, high-quality sources of proteins ensure adequate and excellent sources of these important nutrients.

Controlling Blood Sugar

Research has suggested a link between poor blood sugar levels and brain diseases such as Alzheimer's disease, Parkinson's disease, or dementia. Some factors contributing to Alzheimer's disease may include:

- Enormous intake of carbohydrates, especially from fructose—which is drastically reduced on the ketogenic diet.

- Lack of nutritional fats and good cholesterol — which are copious and healthy on the keto diet

The keto diet helps control blood sugar and improve nutrition; which in turn not only improves insulin response and resistance but also protects against memory loss which is often a part of aging.

Ketogenic Diet and Menopause

There comes an age in a woman's life where her menstrual cycle will finally end. This is when your ovaries stop releasing eggs, better known as ovulation, and therefore menstruation ends. This condition is generally observed in women above the age of 50. There is no defined age that shows when a woman can expect menopause.

There are times where women may experience menopause prematurely as well. This happens if a woman has undergone surgeries like hysterectomy (surgery that involves the removal of ovaries). It can also happen from any injuries that may have caused damage to the ovaries. If this happens before the age of 50, it is classified as premature menopause.

Menopause, as harmless as it sounds, can be quite a troubling phase for women. The hot flashes you experience will keep you up at night, with an elevated heartbeat. The constant feeling of being irritated and a clear downfall in your sex life can contribute greatly towards you feeling more and more grumpy.

Menopause takes a toll on your hormonal balance and the newly developed imbalance then pushes your body to gain massive weight, experience mood swings like never before, and a libido that is crashing faster than you can imagine.

If you think this is bad, here are some other issues that menopause can lead to:

- Chronic stress
- Anxiety
- Insulin spike
- Type 2 diabetes
- Heart diseases
- Polycystic Ovarian Syndrome (PCOS)

The overall picture, then, is grim! Fortunately, a difference in lifestyle and a carefully thought-out diet plan can change all that for you. I am not saying it happens overnight or within a week, but the profound impacts are felt rather quick. In the longer run, keto will rescue you and your body from impending doom and allow you to lead a life without worrying about keeping a glucose monitor or any of the typical health-related equipment near you.

The keto diet, while there are many classes of it, helps your hormones be balanced. This means that you do not have to worry about insulin or any other hormones, hence minimizing the hot flashes and other symptoms. Even if they occur, they will be minor and far less painful.

Moreover, the keto diet jump-starts your sex drive. The fat-rich diet improves fat-soluble vitamin absorption. Not to forget, it especially helps with vitamin D, a vital micronutrient that goes missing with age. All in all, this provides all the drive you need to have intimate moments even in your fifties.

Heart Diseases

Keto diets help women over 50 to shed those extra pounds. Reducing any amount of weight greatly reduces the chances of a heart attack or any other heart complications. Through a carefully selected diet routine, not only are you losing weight and enjoying scrumptious meals, but you are significantly boosting your heart's health and reviving yourself from the otherwise dull state that you may have been in before.

Diabetes Control

Needless to say, the careful selection of ingredients, when cooked together, provide nutrition that is free from any processed or harmful contents such as sugar. Add this to that the fact that keto automatically controls your insulin levels. The result is a glucose level that is always under control and continued control would lead to a day where you will say goodbye to the medications you might be taking for diabetes.

And so Much More!

By taking up the challenge and adapting the keto way, you are ensuring yourself one of the safest journeys into the older years, if not the safest of the lot. Sure, there will be days where you may miss a type of food or two, but that craving will be overshadowed by the benefits the keto diet will bring you.

With the help of the keto diet, you can expect a few more benefits such as:

- Improved and stable blood pressure levels

- A deeper sleep for those suffering from insomnia
- Improved kidney function
- More energy that lasts all day
- Improved bodily functions

Most Common Mistakes and How to Fix Them

1 - Not Getting Enough Magnesium, Potassium, And Sodium

Usually, a regular diet contains plenty of sodium because most processed food contains high amounts of salt. The majority of people find that when they go keto and cut processed foods, they are low on it.

You may not think of low sodium as an issue, but this usually leads to fatigue and cravings.

Potassium is sometimes more lacking while you are on a ketogenic diet, so make sure you get enough of it, especially if you're an active person. Eating spinach and avocados can help you with this.

Lastly, magnesium is a mineral that many of us initially lack. Many people point to the degradation of the soil as a possible explanation for our widespread nutritional shortcomings. Magnesium is essential for sleep, mood, muscles, and general well-being, so it is also good to ensure that you get enough of it. Drinking bone broth is an excellent way to add more of these minerals to your ketogenic diet – it contains sodium, potassium, and magnesium.

2 Not Eating Enough Greens

The key to a ketogenic diet is eating fewer carbohydrates. Many people think that this means avoiding all vegetables. Do not do that, please.

It's true that growing vegetables, such as onions or mushrooms, contain a reasonable amount of carbohydrates, so you may want to limit them, however, eating a lot of vegetables is essential to ensure you get plenty of vitamins and minerals. There are several ways you can incorporate more vegetables into your diet. Salads, sauces, and green smoothies are all quick and easy to make.

3 Not Training

It can be tough to stick to keto in the first few weeks, and it feels terrible to go to the gym. However, if you can manage it, it is reasonable to try to do some exercise. Often, it will help you get keto-adapted faster and help you lose fat (as opposed to muscle).

Walking is one of the most natural options, but at home, you should also do bodyweight exercises such as push-ups, sit-ups, and squats.

How long do I have to stay on keto?

There's no fixed rule on how long a ketogenic diet will last.

Many keto dieters see it as an aid to weight loss or mental clarity. Some are going to have a ketogenic diet for several weeks, and others can have a few months of the paleo diet and then go back to a ketogenic diet again.

However, if you use a ketogenic diet for medicinal reasons, you may need to remain on it for longer – this is something to speak to a health professional about.

Chapter 3. Intermittent Fasting and Keto Diet

What Is Intermittent Fasting?

Much like the ketogenic diet, intermittent fasting (IF) is picking up more popularity by the year! IF is an eating pattern you are going to follow which has periods of fasting and periods of eating. When you eat in this manner, you will be focusing on the foods allowed on the ketogenic diet, along with deciding when you are going to eat them.

Fasting has been practiced since time immemorial. When you think about it, our ancestors did not have food available year-round. When they were unable to find food, they had to learn how to function without food for extended periods of time. In the modern world, we have a McDonald's at every corner, which is both a blessing and a curse! For this reason, fasting is actually much more natural for us compared to eating three or even four meals in a day!

How Does It Work?

If this is your first time trying the ketogenic diet, you may want to wait to incorporate this style of eating. It is going to be enough work figuring out what you are allowed to eat on the ketogenic diet. When you are ready, there are several types of intermittent fasting that you can try out. Much like with our diets, everyone is allowed to be on a different schedule. What works for you may not work for your friend! But this is one of the best parts of the diet; it is completely customizable to your needs!

16/8 Method

This first popular method is known as the Lean gains Protocol. For this method, you will skip breakfast and only eat for eight hours during the day. An example of this could be 12-8 p.m. Once those hours are up, you would then fast for sixteen hours. During your fast, you eat nothing or very little amounts of food if you are desperate.

5:2 Diet

This next method is a bit different compared to typical fasting. For the 5:2 diet, you spend two days eating only 500-600 calories. On the rest of the days, you are allowed to eat normally.

Eat-Stop-Eat

The Eat-Stop-Eat fasting method involves not eating for 24 hours straight for one or two days a week. For the other days, you are allowed to eat normally.

Crescendo Method

For women over 50, this may be your best option. For the Crescendo Method, you will only be fasting for 12-16 hours for 2-3 days a week. These days of fasting should be nonconsecutive and spaced throughout your week. For example, you would want to fast for Monday, Wednesday, and again on Friday.

Intermittent fasting works because, during these fasts, you are reducing your overall calorie intake for the week. The fewer calories you consume, the more weight you are going to lose. For this reason, you need to make sure you are not compensating for this calorie reduction by overeating during the times you are allowed to eat. It is all about moderation and finding a good balance in your diet.

Intermittent Fasting and Hormones

As you follow the ketogenic diet combined with intermittent fasting, there are several things that will be happening to you on a molecular and cellular level. One of the major benefits being that as you fast, your body will adjust your hormone levels to make your body fat more accessible. This is beneficial on the ketogenic diet because you are now using the fat as energy anyway!

Fasting also initiates cellular repair within your body. This process is known as autophagy. During autophagy, your cells begin to digest and remove any dysfunctional proteins that are old and built inside your cells. Fasting also helps promote proper gene expression that may help protect against disease and help you live a longer and healthier life!

What's the Benefit for Weight Loss?

If you are looking to lose weight on the ketogenic diet, it will be beneficial for you to pair it with Intermittent Fasting. With this manner of eating, you will be eating fewer meals and reducing your number of calories automatically. Once this is complete, your body will begin lowering the insulin in your system and increase the fat-burning hormones in your system. This meaning that through short-term fasting, you can increase your metabolic rate and get rid of excess weight!

Health Benefits of Intermittent Fasting

While weight loss is an incredible benefit in itself, intermittent fasting will offer you several other benefits as well. Some of the other benefits include:

- Decreased inflammation
- Improved heart health
- Increased brain health
- Increased life span

Intermittent fasting can also help you to lead a simpler lifestyle. When you are eating three to four meals a day, this requires a lot of time to cook and plan healthy meals. When you are only eating for a certain amount of time, this gives you more time to do the things that you want without worrying about fitting a meal in!

Intermittent Fasting on the Keto Diet

Here are some of the core reasons why you should combine an IF program with your ketogenic diet.

- It will help you to purge cancerous and pre-cancerous cells.
- It will greatly accelerate the process of fat-burning.

- It will enhance your gene expression and give you a longer lifespan.
- It will encourage cellular clearing and repairing.
- It will improve your insulin sensitivity.
- It will decrease oxidative stress and inflammation.
- It will help you enhance your cognitive effects and protect your brain.
- It will help you to stabilize your blood sugar levels.

Aside from the above-mentioned points, two more factors should be taken into consideration, which will vastly benefit your ketogenic regime.

It will help you to enter ketosis sooner: since the ketogenic diet is carefully designed to push your body into ketosis and forces it to run on ketones from the low carb intake, you are already fasting yourself of glucose and carbs.

This actually mimics the fasting state that comes from intermittent fasting.

That being said, if you combine your carbohydrate fast with an IF regimen, then the time period required for you to enter ketosis will be significantly decreased.

It will help you to avoid the side effects that arise from ketosis. If you are completely new to the ketogenic diet and are trying it out for the first time, then you might experience some minor side effects.

However, if you combine your ketogenic diet with an IF program, then side effects such as keto flu are greatly reduced!

Not to mention the fact that your low-carb diet will make it much easier for you to fast since your body will be running on ketones rather than carbs.

A Note on Weight Loss

Perhaps one of the biggest reasons people tend to pursue IF is for weight loss.

The ketogenic diet will help you to lose weight but combining both of the programs will help you to lose even more.

Our bodies are designed to take only a certain number of calories in one go. So, limiting your food intake windows will greatly decrease the number of calories that you are ingesting, leading to an accelerated weight loss when combined with a ketogenic diet.

Since you will be fasting most of the time, it will help you to eliminate unnecessary snacking.

The high-fat keto diet alongside the body's ketosis effect will help you reduce your appetite and increase satiety levels. This will greatly help you to fast comfortably since your body won't be craving snacks or food.

Tips for Keto Fasting

Always make sure to eat plenty: IF will naturally help you to eat less, but when you are in your non-fasting window, make sure to eat a good amount of nutritious, ketogenic food, maintain your ketogenic macros and calorie intake, and avoid any metabolic issues.

Try to measure your ketone levels and keep track of them. Fasting will almost definitely help you to stay in ketosis for a prolonged period of time, but it is important to make sure that you are not eating too much protein or carbs during non-fasting periods that might kick you out of ketosis. Therefore, it is a good practice to keep your ketosis in check.

Intermittent Fasting for Seniors

There are some diseases or health-related issues that are more prevalent in women over 50, and in this section, we will look at these and how they are affected by intermittent fasting.

Some of the diseases or health-related issues that are more likely to affect women over the age of 50 include joint pain, arthritis, lower metabolism (which can lead to weight gain), reduced muscle mass, sleep disturbances, increased levels of belly fat, osteoporosis and other common but weight and age-related diseases such as heart disease or diabetes. By practicing intermittent fasting and losing weight, you will reduce your risk of developing several of these diseases. By inducing autophagy, you are reducing your risk of those diseases that are not as closely related to weight, such as cancer and heart attacks.

Joint Health

In women over 50, there is a higher risk of developing joint issues such as pain of the knees, wrists, elbows, or shoulders. This is due to an increase in age and a higher risk of arthritis or lower back and other joint pain due to overuse. In studies where women over 50 practiced intermittent fasting for a period of time, decreased levels of joint pain, arthritic symptoms, and lower back pain were found.

How Women Over 50 Can Benefit from Intermittent Fasting

As you have seen evidenced up until now, intermittent fasting is extremely beneficial for women over 50, and most of the research done around this type of diet regime points to positive effects. It is quite difficult to find research that doesn't support intermittent fasting for women over 50 as an effective tool for weight loss, improved health, and better overall mental health. As long as intermittent fasting is followed in a safe manner, the results can be extremely positive!

Things for Women Over 50 to Keep in Mind

Supplementing may be very beneficial and even necessary when fasting to maintain and improve health. Some essential nutrients and minerals that your body would greatly benefit from, like Omega-3 or iron, may be difficult to get in adequate amounts if you are fasting. For this reason, supplementing them may benefit you in terms of keeping you feeling healthy and energetic, as well as keeping your brain functioning to its full potential. You can take specific nutrients on their own in pill-form or you can opt for a multivitamin that will include all of the most essential vitamins and minerals for overall good health. These vitamins and minerals may differ from those that we looked at previously, which included vitamins and minerals that are known to induce autophagy. The vitamins included in a multivitamin will be those that are known to promote good overall health and which are usually obtained through a balanced, whole food diet.

Nutrients You Need and How to Get Them

In this section, we are going to look at the most beneficial nutrients for your body and where/ how you can find them when following a specific diet. For women over the age of 50, it is important to ensure that you are getting all of the nutrients that your body needs, especially if you are trying to lose weight or are following a regime that includes fasting. To ensure that during your fasting periods, you are as healthy as possible, supplementation is something that could be considered, to ensure that you are feeding your body the nutrients it needs. It is always preferable to get the nutrients you need from whole foods rather than from supplements, but in some cases, when you cannot get everything you need from the foods in your diet alone (especially if you are eating fewer calories), then supplementation is always better than nothing. Below, we will look at some whole food sources as well as some supplements that you may wish to consider.

Omega-3 Fatty Acids

These are essential since they cannot be made in our bodies. Omega-3 fatty acids are substances that are necessary to get from your diet as the body cannot make them on its own. These fatty acids are the most essential and the most beneficial for our brains and bodies in general. They have numerous effects on the brain including reducing inflammation (which reduces the risk of Alzheimer's) and maintaining and improving mood and cognitive function, including memory. Omega-3 fatty acids have these great beneficial effects because of the way that they act in the brain, which is what makes them so essential to our diets. Omega-3 fatty acids increase the production of new nerve cells in the brain by acting specifically on the nerve stem cells within the brain, causing new and healthy nerve cells to be generated.

Omega-3 fatty acids can be found in fish like salmon, sardines, black cod, and herring. It can also be taken in pill form for those who do not eat fish or cannot eat enough of it. It can also be taken in the form of a fish oil supplement like krill oil.

Omega-3 is by far the most important nutrient that you need because of the numerous benefits that come from it, for both the brain and the body. While supplements are often the last step when it comes to trying to include something in your diet, for Omega-3's the benefits are too great to potentially miss by trying to receive all of it from your diet.

Sulphoraphane

What do brussels sprouts, cabbage, kale, broccoli, and sprouts have in common? All of these green vegetables have one thing in common- they all contain sulforaphane. Sulforaphane is a plant chemical found naturally in these vegetables. This is an antioxidant that acts in a similar way to turmeric and thus has similar benefits. Sulforaphane, like turmeric, induces autophagy in the brain which helps to reduce the risk of Alzheimer's, Parkinson's, and dementia which are all neurodegenerative diseases. Neurodegeneration means that the cells in the brain (called nerves) are damaged and break down which leads to cognitive decline like in Alzheimer's or physical decline as in Parkinson's. These vegetables can help to treat these diseases by slowing their progression, as they are all diseases that come about over time. There is no cure yet, but the treatment at this stage involves delaying the progression of these diseases.

Sulforaphane can be found in the aforementioned vegetables, but the strongest source are broccoli and sprouts. It can also be taken concentrated in a supplement form.

Calcium

Calcium is beneficial for the healthy circulation of blood, and for maintaining strong bones and teeth. Calcium can come from dairy products like milk, yogurt, and cheese. It can also be found in leafy greens like kale, broccoli and sardines.

Magnesium

Magnesium is beneficial for your diet as it also helps you to maintain strong bones and teeth. Magnesium and calcium are most effective when ingested together, as magnesium helps in the absorption of calcium. It also helps to reduce migraines and is great for relieving stress and anxiety. Magnesium can be found in leafy green vegetables like kale and spinach, as well as fruits like bananas and raspberries, legumes like beans and chickpeas, vegetables like peas, cabbage, green beans, asparagus, and brussels sprouts, and fish like tuna and salmon.

Exogenous Ketones

When tested on animal models, even when they were ingested on a normal carbohydrate intake diet, these exogenous ketones proved to be beneficial in terms of helping the models with problems like seizures, targeting cancer, inflammation, and anxiety. These are diseases that we normally see to be assisted by ketosis (which is the state the body enters when it is using fat as a source of fuel instead of carbohydrates).

Electrolytes

When you first begin following an intermittent fasting regime, having electrolyte depletion is quite common. This is because of water weight loss occurs through lower carbohydrate intake. Taking electrolyte supplements can help to avoid a deficiency in common electrolytes, like magnesium, potassium, and sodium. This is also why you should ensure you are getting enough dietary sodium, as this is an electrolyte that you need. Along with this, though, you will need to ensure you are drinking enough water to avoid dehydration.

Iron

This one is a little tricky, but it is worth noting. Iron should be obtained in the right amounts in your diet through whole foods. If you feel like you might be deficient in iron and you are having trouble getting it in the foods you eat, you can visit your doctor for advice on this topic. Iron cannot be supplemented without being referred by a doctor first, as it is something that they would like you to first try to get from your food. If this is becoming a problem, they can give you supplements to take. This is especially a concern if you are not eating much red meat, and this may lead your doctor to want you to begin supplementing. Make an appointment with your doctor to find out more about this topic.

Vitamin D

Vitamin D is found in some foods that have been fortified with it, but in a natural sense, it can be found in only a few foods. These include cheese, fatty fish like salmon and tuna, as well as egg yolks. Another source are organic mushrooms that have been exposed to UV rays.

Vitamin D can be absorbed naturally through sun exposure, so if you live in a sunny place, make sure you get hour, for some walks or some timer with the sun on your skin. If you live in a colder or gloomier place, consider purchasing a lamp that mimics the sun and provides you with vitamin D in your house. On a sunny day in cold weather, getting sun on your face will give you vitamin D.

This one is something that everyone should be conscious of, but it is especially necessary to examine if you are following a specific diet.

Bioactive Compounds

Bioactive compounds are compounds found within foods that act in the body in beneficial ways. The bioactive compounds found within berries, such as acai berries, strawberries, and blueberries are very beneficial for your health. The bioactive compounds in these specific berries work in the brain to induce autophagy and reduce inflammation. This leads to the protection of brain cells in this case from oxidative stress. Oxidative stress is something that can happen within the brain when there is an imbalance of oxygen, which can cause reduced cognitive functioning. These berries and their induction of autophagy helps to reduce this by keeping the balance of oxygen at a healthy level.

Risks of Intermittent Fasting

With those benefits in mind, it should be stated that intermittent fasting is not for everyone. For example, if you are underweight or have a history of eating disorders, you will want to consult with a professional before you begin intermittent fasting or the ketogenic diet. With these two methods combined, your diet will be doing you more harm than good.

It should be noted that there are also some side-effects you can expect in intermittent fasting. One of the major symptoms will be hunger. Up until this point, your body has been used to be provided with food all day long. When you take this away, you will probably get hungry. You may also feel weak at times, but these symptoms should go away once your body adapts to the new schedule.

You will also want to consult with a professional if you have any of the following:

- Pregnant or breastfeeding
- History of amenorrhea
- Trying to get pregnant
- Take medications
- Have low blood pressure or problems with blood sugar regulation
- Have diabetes

Chapter 4. Keto Recipes

Breakfast Recipes

1 French Omelet

Preparation Time: 10 minutes

Cooking Time: 10 minutes

Servings: 2

Ingredients:

2 large eggs

4 egg whites

¼ cup of milk

1/8 tsp of pepper

1/8 tsp of salt

1 cup of ham (cooked)

1 tbsp of green pepper (chopped)

1 tbsp of onion (chopped)

1/2 cup of cheddar cheese (shredded)

Directions

Whisk the first five listed ingredients.

Use a cooking spray for greasing a skillet. Place the skillet over medium flame. Add the mixture of eggs.

Cook for two minutes.

Top with the remaining ingredients. Fold the egg in half.

Cut the omelet in half. Serve immediately.

Nutrition: Calories: 189; Protein: 22.3 g; Carbs: 3.6 g; Fat: 10.9 g; Fiber: 0.1 g

2 Sage Sausage Patty

Preparation Time: 10 minutes

Cooking Time: 10 hours 10 minutes

Servings: 8

Ingredients:

1 lb pork (ground)

3/4 cup cheddar cheese (ground)

1/4 cup buttermilk

1 tbsp onion (chopped)

2 tsp sage

3/4 tsp pepper

3/4 tsp salt

½ tsp oregano (dried)

½ tsp garlic powder

Directions:

Combine the listed ingredients either in a bowl or in a food processor.

Shape the mixture into eight equal patties of half-inch thickness. Refrigerate the patties for one hour.

Heat oil in an iron skillet. Cook the patties on each side for six minutes.

Serve hot.

Nutrition: Calories: 160.3; Protein: 14.6 g; Carbs: 1.2 g; Fat: 12.3 g; Fiber: 0.3 g

3 Feta Frittata

Preparation Time: 15 minutes

Cooking Time: 15 minutes

Servings: 2

Ingredients:

1 green onion (sliced)

1 clove of garlic (minced)

2 large eggs

½ cup egg substitute

4 tbsps feta cheese (crumbled)

1/3 cup plum tomato (chopped)

4 slices avocado (peeled)

2 tbsp sour cream

Directions:

Heat oil in an iron skillet. Add garlic and onion. Sauté for three minutes.

Combine egg substitute, eggs, and three tablespoons of feta cheese in a bowl. Add the egg mixture to the skillet.

Cook for six minutes.

Sprinkle remaining feta and tomato on top.

Cover and cook for two minutes.

Let the egg rest for five minutes.

Serve with sour cream and avocado.

Nutrition Facts: Calories: 205.3; Protein: 19.3 g; Carbs: 6.7 g; Fat: 12.5 g; Fiber: 3.6 g

4 Ham Steak with Bacon, Mushrooms, and Gruyere

Preparation Time: 25 minutes

Cooking Time: 10 minutes

Servings: 4

Ingredients:

2 tbsp butter

½ lb mushrooms (sliced)

1 shallot (chopped)

2 cloves garlic (minced)

1/8 tsp black pepper (ground)

1 boneless ham steak (cooked, cut in four equal pieces)

1 cup gruyere cheese (shredded)

4 strips bacon (cooked, crumbled)

1 tbsp parsley (minced)

Directions:

Heat butter in a large iron skillet. Add shallot and mushrooms. Cook the mixture for six minutes. Mix garlic and pepper. Sauté for two minutes. Keep aside.

Cook the ham in the same skillet. Add bacon and cheese. Cook for two minutes.

Serve the ham with the mushroom mixture from the top.

Nutrition: Calories: 356.3; Protein: 35.4 g; Carbs: 5.1 g; Fat: 23.2 g; Fiber: 1.1 g

5 Mushroom-Mascarpone Frittata

Preparation Time: 25 minutes

Cooking Time: 20 minutes

Servings: 6

Ingredients:

8 large eggs

1/3 cup of whipping cream

1/2 cup of Romano cheese (grated)

2 tsp salt

5 tbsp olive oil

¾ lb fresh mushrooms (sliced)

1 onion (sliced)

2 tbsp basil (minced)

2 cloves garlic (minced)

1/8 tsp of pepper

8 oz of mascarpone cheese

Directions:

Whisk together cream, eggs, one-fourth cup of Romano cheese, and salt in a bowl.

Heat two tablespoons of oil in a pan. Add mushrooms and onion. Sauté for two minutes. Add garlic, basil, along with pepper. Stir for one minute. Remove from heat. Add Romano cheese and mascarpone cheese.

Heat one tablespoon of oil in the same pan. Add half mixture of eggs to the pan. Keep cooking for seven minutes. Repeat with the remaining egg mixture.

Place one egg frittata on a plate. Add the mixture of mushrooms. Spread properly.

Add the other layer of the frittata.

Cut in wedges.

Serve immediately.

Nutrition: Calories: 469.3 | Protein: 18.7 g | Carbs: 5.7 g| Fat: 45.4 g | Fiber: 1.6 g

6   Broccoli Quiche Cups

Preparation Time: 5 minutes

Cooking Time: 20 minutes

Servings: 6

Ingredients:

1 cup broccoli (chopped)

1½ cup pepper jack cheese (shredded)

6 large eggs

¾ cup whipping cream

½ cup of bacon bits

1 shallot (minced)

¼ tsp of pepper

¼ tsp of salt

Directions:

Preheat your oven at one-hundred and 70°C.

Divide the cheese and chopped broccoli among twelve greased muffin cups.

Combine the remaining ingredients in a bowl. Divide the prepared mixture among the cups.

Bake the quiche cups for twenty minutes.

Serve immediately.

Nutrition: Calories: 292.3; Protein: 17.6 g; Carbs: 3.6 g; Fat: 25.4 g; Fiber: 0.7 g

7 Savory Chicken Sausage-Apple

Preparation Time: 10 minutes

Cooking Time: 15 minutes

Servings: 4

Ingredients:

1 tart apple (peeled, diced)

2 tsp poultry seasoning

1 tsp salt

¼ tsp of pepper

1 lb chicken (ground)

Directions:

Take a large bowl. Mix the first four ingredients. Crumble the chicken over the apple mixture. Combine well. Shape the mixture into eight equal patties of three-inch thickness.

Heat oil in an iron skillet.

Cook the apple-chicken patties for six minutes on each side.

Serve hot.

Nutrition: Calories: 93.6; Protein: 9.9 g; Carbs: 3.2 g; Fat: 6.5 g; Fiber: 1.2 g

8 Manchego and Shiitake Scramble

Preparation Time: 10 minutes

Cooking Time: 15 minutes

Servings: 8

Ingredients:

2 tbsp olive oil

½ cup sweet red pepper (diced)

1/2 cup onion (diced)

2 cups shiitake mushrooms (sliced)

1 tsp prepared horseradish

8 large eggs (beaten)

1 cup whipping cream

1 cup of Manchego cheese (shredded)

½ tsp of pepper (ground)

½ tsp of kosher salt

Directions:

Heat one tablespoon of oil in an iron skillet. Add red pepper and onion. Cook for three minutes. Cook the mixture for four minutes after adding the mushrooms along with horseradish. Stir for two minutes.

Whisk the remaining ingredients in a bowl with some olive oil. Pour the mixture into the skillet.

Cook and scramble the eggs for four minutes.

Serve hot.

Nutrition: Calories: 143 Cal; Fat: 11.23 g; Protein: 7.22 g; Carbs: 3.34 g

9 Three-Cheese Quiche

Preparation Time: 10 minutes

Cooking Time: 1 hour

Servings: 6

Ingredients:

7 large eggs

5 egg yolks

1 cup of whipping cream

1 cup of half and half cream

1 cup of mozzarella cheese (shredded)

¾ cup of cheddar cheese (shredded)

½ cup of Swiss cheese (shredded)

2 tbsp of sun-dried tomatoes

1½ tsp of seasoning blend

¼ tsp of basil (dried)

Directions:

Preheat your oven at 150°C.

Combine egg yolks, eggs, whipping cream, mozzarella cheese, half and half cream, half cup of cheddar cheese, tomatoes, Swiss cheese, basil, and seasoning blend in a greased pie dish. Sprinkle the remaining cheddar cheese on the top.

Bake for 50 minutes.

Let the quiche sit for 10 minutes.

Cut in triangles and serve.

Nutrition: Calories: 448.3; Protein: 21.2 g; Carbs: 5.2 g; Fat: 38.6 g; Fiber: 0.2 g

Breakfast Turkey Sausage

Preparation Time: 10 minutes

Cooking Time: 12 minutes

Servings: 8

Ingredients:

1 lb lean turkey (ground)

¾ tsp salt

½ tsp rubbed sage

¼ tsp ginger (ground)

1/3 tsp pepper (ground)

Directions:

Crumble the turkey meat in a large bowl. Add sage, salt, ginger, and pepper. Shape the mixture into eight equal patties of two-inch thickness.

Grease an iron skillet with oil.

Add the patties. Cook for six minutes on each side.

Nutrition Facts: Calories: 87.6; Protein: 11.3 g; Carbs: 0.2 g; Fat: 7.5 g; Fiber: 0.1 g

11 No-Bread Breakfast Sandwich

Preparation Time: 7 minutes

Cooking Time: 8 minutes

Servings: 2

Ingredients:

2 tbsp butter

4 large eggs

Pepper and salt

1 oz deli ham (smoked)

2 oz cheddar cheese (cut in slices)

Few drops of Tabasco

Directions:

Heat the butter in an iron skillet. Add the eggs. Fry each side for two minutes. Add pepper and salt.

Take a fried egg. Add ham and cheese. Top with another fried egg.

Repeat for the other fried eggs.

Place the sandwich in the pan for one minute.

Sprinkle some Tabasco on top.

Serve hot.

Nutrition: Calories: 356.3; Protein: 20.3 g; Carbs: 2.1 g; Fat: 31.1 g; Fiber: 0.2 g

12 Baked Eggs

Preparation Time: 5 minutes

Cooking Time: 15 minutes

Servings: 1

Ingredients:

3 oz beef (ground)

2 large eggs

2 oz of cheese (shredded)

Directions:

Preheat your oven at 200°C.

Arrange the ground beef as the base in a baking dish.

Make two holes in the beef base. Crack the eggs in the holes.

Sprinkle cheese on top.

Bake for 15 minutes.

Let the baked eggs rest for 5 minutes.

Nutrition Facts: Calories: 497.6; Protein: 42.1 g; Carbs: 2.1 g; Fat: 34.5 g; Fiber: 0.3 g

13 Cured Salmon with Chives and Scrambled Eggs

Preparation Time: 7 minutes

Cooking Time: 8 minutes

Servings: 2

Ingredients:

2 large eggs

2 tbsp butter

¼ cup whipping cream

1 tbsp chives (chopped)

2 oz cured salmon

Pepper and salt

Directions:

Begin with whisking the eggs in a bowl.

Heat the butter in a pan. Add the eggs. Add the cream. Stir for three minutes.

Simmer for five minutes. Keep stirring to makw the eggs creamy.

Add salt, chopped chives, and pepper.

Serve the eggs with cured salmon.

Nutrition Facts: Calories: 730.2; Protein: 49.6 g; Carbs: 2.1 g; Fat: 61.3 g; Fiber: 0.1 g

Eggs Benedict on Avocados

Preparation Time: 10 minutes

Cooking Time: 10 minutes

Servings: 4

Ingredients:

For the hollandaise:

3 egg yolks

1 tbsp of lemon juice

Pepper and salt

8 tbsp of butter (unsalted)

For the eggs:

2 avocados (pitted, skinned)

4 large eggs

5 oz salmon (smoked)

Directions:

Add the butter to a bowl. Microwave for twenty seconds.

Add lemon juice and egg yolks. Use a hand blender for properly blending the mixture. Keep blending until a white layer forms. Add pepper and salt. Blend for two minutes.

Boil water in a saucepan. Crack the eggs in a small cup by cracking one egg at a time. Slide the eggs gently into the water. Cook for four minutes.

Cut the avocados in half. Add an egg on top of each avocado slice. Add hollandaise sauce on top.

Add smoked salmon as the side.

Serve immediately.

Nutrition Facts: Calories: 523.6; Protein: 17.6 g; Carbs: 3.1 g; Fat: 49.3 g; Fiber: 7.1 g

15   Keto Chaffles

Preparation Time: 4 minutes

Cooking Time: 6 minutes

Servings: 4

Ingredients:

1 oz butter (melted)

4 large eggs

8 oz of mozzarella cheese (shredded)

4 tbsp of almond flour

A pinch of salt

Directions:

Preheat a waffle maker.

Mix all the ingredients that have been listed in a mixing bowl. Combine well.

Use butter to grease the waffle maker.

Add one spoonful of the batter to the waffle maker. Close the waffle maker. Cook for six minutes.

Serve immediately with toppings of your choice.

Nutrition: Calories: 332.3; Protein: 23.2 g; Carbs: 1.9 g; Fat: 28.6 g; Fiber: 0.2 g

Lunch Recipes

1 Melt-in-Your-Mouth Ribs

Preparation Time: 30 minutes

Cooking Time: 4 hours

Servings: 4

Ingredients:

1½ lb spare ribs

1 tbsp olive oil, at room temperature

2 cloves garlic, chopped

1 Italian pepper, chopped

Salt and black peppercorns to taste

½ tsp ground cumin

2 bay leaves

A bunch of green onions, chopped

¾ cup beef bone broth, preferably homemade

2 tsp erythritol

Directions:

Heat the olive oil in a saucepan over medium-high heat. Sear the ribs for 6-7 minutes on each side.

Whisk the broth, erythritol, garlic, Italian pepper, green onions, salt, pepper, and cumin until well combined.

Place the spare ribs in your crockpot; pour in the pepper/broth mixture. Add in the bay leaves. Cook for about 4 hours on the low setting.

Storage

Divide the pork ribs into four portions. Place each portion of ribs along with the cooking juices in an airtight container; store in your refrigerator for 3-5 days.

To freeze, place the ribs in airtight containers or heavy-duty freezer bags. Freeze for up to 4 to 6 months. Defrost in the refrigerator. Reheat in your oven at 250°F until heated through. Bon appétit!

Nutrition: 412 Calories; 14 g Fat; 4.3 g Carbs; 43.3 g Protein; 0.7 g Fiber

2 Mom's Meatballs in Creamy Sauce

Preparation Time: 5 minutes

Cooking Time: 25 minutes

Servings: 6

Ingredients:

For the Meatballs:

2 eggs

1 tbsp steak seasoning

1 tbsp green garlic, minced

1 tbsp scallions, minced

1 lb ground pork

1/2 lb ground turkey

For the Sauce:

3 tsp ghee

1 cup double cream

1 cup cream of onion soup

Salt and pepper to your liking

½ tsp dried rosemary

Directions:

Preheat your oven to 365°F.

In a mixing bowl, combine all ingredients for the meatballs. Roll the mixture into 20 to 24 balls and place them on a parchment-lined baking sheet.

Roast for about 25 minutes or until your meatballs are golden-brown on the top.

While your meatballs are roasting, melt the ghee in a preheated sauté pan over a moderate flame. Gradually add in the remaining ingredients, whisking constantly, until the sauce has reduced slightly.

Storage

Place the meatballs along with the sauce in airtight containers or Ziploc bags; keep in your refrigerator for up to 3-4 days.

Freeze the meatballs in the sauce in airtight containers or heavy-duty freezer bags. Freeze for up to 3-4 months. Reheat on the stove pot or in your oven. Bon appétit!

Nutrition: 378 Calories; 29.9 g Fat; 2.9 g Carbs; 23.4 g Protein; 0.3 g Fiber

3 Mexican-Style Pork Chops

Preparation Time: 15 minutes

Cooking Time: 30 minutes

Servings: 6

Ingredients:

2 Mexican chilies, chopped

1 tsp dried Mexican oregano

½ tsp red pepper flakes, crushed

Salt and ground black pepper, to taste

6 pork chops

½ cup chicken stock

2 garlic cloves, minced

2 tbsp vegetable oil

Directions:

Heat 1 tablespoon of the olive oil in a frying pan over moderate to high heat. Brow the pork chops for 5-6 minutes per side.

Then, bring the Mexican chilies and chicken stock to a boil; remove from the heat and let it sit for about 20 minutes.

Puree the chilies along with the liquid and the remaining ingredients in your food processor. Add in the remaining oil.

Storage

Divide the pork chops and sauce into six portions; place each portion in a separate airtight container or Ziploc bag; keep in your refrigerator for 3-4 days.

Freeze the pork chops in sauce in airtight containers or heavy-duty freezer bags. Freeze for up to 4 months. Defrost in the refrigerator and reheat in a saucepan. Bon appétit!

Nutrition: 356 Calories; 20.3 g Fat; 0.3 g Carbs; 45.2 g Protein; 0 g Fiber

4 Easy Pork Tenderloin Gumbo

Preparation Time: 15 minutes

Cooking Time: 35 minutes

Servings: 6

Ingredients:

1 lb pork tenderloin, cubed

8 oz New Orleans spicy sausage, sliced

1 tbsp Cajun spice mix

1 medium-sized leek, chopped

2 tbsp olive oil

5 cups bone broth

½ cup celery, chopped

1 tsp gumbo file

¼ cup flaxseed meal

¾ lb okra

2 bell peppers, de-veined and thinly sliced

Directions:

In a heavy-bottomed pot, heat the oil until sizzling. Sear the pork tenderloin and New Orleans sausage for about 8 minutes or until browned on all sides; set aside.

In the same pot, cook the leek and peppers until they softened. Add in the gumbo file, Cajun spice, and broth. Bring it to a rolling boil.

Turn the heat to medium-low and add in celery. Let it simmer for 18-20 minutes.

Stir in the flaxseed meal and okra along with the reserved meat. Then, continue to simmer for 5-6 minutes or until heated through.

Storage

Spoon your gumbo into six airtight containers; keep in your refrigerator for up to 3-4 days.

For freezing, place the chilled gumbo in airtight containers or heavy-duty freezer bags. Freeze for up to 5 months. Defrost in the refrigerator and reheat on the stove pot. Enjoy!

Nutrition: 427 Calories; 16.2 g Fat; 3.6 g Carbs; 33.2 g Protein; 4.4 g Fiber

5 Pork and Carrot Mini Muffins

Preparation Time: 15 minutes

Cooking Time: 35 minutes

Servings: 6

Ingredients:

1 egg, whisked

1 oz envelope onion soup mix

Kosher salt and ground black pepper, to taste

2 cloves of garlic, minced

1 cup carrots, shredded

1 cup tomato puree

1 tbsp coconut aminos

1 tbsp stone-ground mustard

1½ tsp dry basil

1 cup Romano cheese, grated

1 lb pork, ground

½ lb turkey, ground

Directions:

In a mixing bowl, combine all ingredients until everything is well incorporated. Press the mixture into a lightly oiled muffin tin.

Bake in the preheated oven at 355°F for 30-33 minutes; let it cool slightly before unmolding and serving.

Storage

Wrap the meatloaf muffins tightly with heavy-duty aluminum foil or plastic wrap. Keep in your refrigerator for up to 3 to 4 days.

For freezing, wrap the meatloaf muffins tightly to prevent freezer burn. They will maintain the best quality for 3-4 months. Defrost in the refrigerator. Bon appétit!

Nutrition: 303 Calories; 17 g Fat; 6.2 g Carbs; 29.6 g Protein; 1.7 g Fiber

6 Bacon Blue Cheese Fat Bombs

Preparation Time: 5 minutes

Cooking Time: 5 minutes

Servings: 4

Ingredients:

1½ tbsp mayonnaise

½ cup bacon, chopped

3 oz blue cheese, crumbled

3 oz cream cheese

2 tbsp chives, chopped

2 tsp tomato puree

Directions:

Mix all ingredients until everything is well combined.

Shape the mixture into 8 equal fat bombs.

Storage

Place the fat bombs in airtight containers or Ziploc bags; keep in your refrigerator for 10 days.

To freeze, arrange the fat bombs on a baking tray in a single layer; freeze for about 2 hours. Transfer the frozen bombs to an airtight container. Freeze for up to 2 months. Serve chilled!

Nutrition: 232 Calories; 17.6 g Fat; 2.9 g Carbs; 14.2 g Protein; 0.6 g Fiber

7 Creole-Style Pork Shank

Preparation Time: 2 hours (marinating time)

Cooking Time: 30 minutes

Servings: 6

Ingredients:

1½ lb pork shank, cut into 6 serving portions

1 tbsp Creole seasoning

A few drops of liquid smoke

Salt and cayenne pepper, to taste

3 tsp vegetable oil

2 clove garlic, minced

1½ tbsp coconut aminos

Directions:

Blend the salt, cayenne pepper, vegetable oil, garlic, liquid smoke, Creole seasoning, and coconut aminos until you get a uniform and creamy mixture.

Massage the pork shanks on all sides with the prepared rub mixture. Let it marinate for about 2 hours in your refrigerator.

Grill for about 20 minutes until cooked through.

Storage

Put the pork shanks into six airtight containers or Ziploc bags; keep in your refrigerator for 3-4 days.

To freeze, wrap tightly with heavy-duty aluminum foil or freezer wrap. It will maintain the best quality for about 3 months. Defrost in the refrigerator and reheat in your oven. Enjoy!

Nutrition: 335 Calories; 24.3 g Fat; 0.8 g Carbs; 26.4 g Protein; 0.4 g Fiber

8 German Pork Rouladen

Preparation Time: 2 hours (marinating time)

Cooking Time: 1 hour

Servings: 6

Ingredients:

1½ lb boneless pork loin, butterflied

2 garlic cloves, pressed

1 tbsp ghee, room temperature

1 tbsp Mediterranean herb mix

1 tsp mustard seeds

½ tsp cumin seeds

1 cup roasted vegetable broth

1 large-sized onion, thinly sliced

Salt and black peppercorns, to taste

½ cup Burgundy wine

Directions:

Boil the pork loin for about 5 minutes; pat it dry.

Now, combine the Mediterranean herb mix, mustard seeds, cumin seeds, garlic, and ghee.

Unfold the pork loin and spread the rub all over the cut side. Roll the pork and secure with kitchen string. Allow it to sit at least 2 hours in your refrigerator.

Place the pork loin in a lightly greased baking pan. Add on wine, broth, onion, salt, and black peppercorns.

Roast in the preheated oven at 390°F for approximately 1 hour.

Storage

Divide the pork and sauce between six airtight containers or Ziploc bags; keep in your refrigerator for up to 3 to 5 days.

For freezing, place the pork and sauce in airtight containers or heavy-duty freezer bags. Freeze for up to 4 months. Defrost in the refrigerator and reheat in your oven. Bon appétit!

Nutrition: 220 Calories; 6 g Fat; 2.8 g Carbs; 33.3 g Protein; 0.4 g Fiber

9 Rich Pork and Bacon Meatloaf

Preparation Time: 20 minutes

Cooking Time: 1 hour 10 minutes

Servings: 6

Ingredients:

1¼ lb ground pork

½ lb pork sausage, broken up

6 strips bacon

2 garlic cloves, finely minced

1 tsp celery seeds

Salt and cayenne pepper, to taste

1 bunch coriander, roughly chopped

1 egg, beaten

2 oz half-and-half

1 tsp lard

1 medium-sized leek, chopped

Directions:

Melt the lard in a frying pan over medium-high heat. Cook the leek and garlic until they have softened or about 3 minutes.

Add in the ground pork and sausage; cook until it is no longer pink, about 3 minutes. Add in the half-and-half, celery seeds, salt, cayenne pepper, coriander, and egg.

Press the mixture into a loaf pan.

Place the bacon strips on top of your meatloaf and bake at 390°F for about 55 minutes.

Storage

Wrap your meatloaf tightly with heavy-duty aluminum foil or plastic wrap. Store in your refrigerator for up to 3-4 days.

For freezing, wrap your meatloaf tightly to prevent freezer burn. Freeze for up to 3-4 months. Defrost in the refrigerator and reheat in your oven. Bon appétit!

Nutrition: 396 Calories; 24.1 g Fat; 5.1 g Carbs; 38.1 g Protein; 0.5 g Fiber

Pork and Vegetable Souvlaki

Preparation Time: 2 hours

Cooking Time: 20 minutes

Servings: 6

Ingredients:

1 tbsp Greek spice mix

2 cloves garlic, crushed

3 tbsp coconut aminos

3 tbsp olive oil

1 tbsp stone-ground mustard

2 tbsp fresh lemon juice

1 lb brown mushrooms

2 bell peppers, cut into thick slices

1 red bell pepper, cut into thick slices

1 zucchini, cubed

1 shallot, cut into wedges

2 lb pork butt, cubed

Bamboo skewers, soaked in cold water for 30 minutes

Directions:

Mix the Greek spice mix, garlic, coconut aminos, olive oil, mustard, and lemon juice in a ceramic dish; add in pork cubes and let it marinate for 2 hours.

Thread the pork cubes and vegetables onto the soaked skewers. Salt to taste.

Grill for about 15 minutes, basting with the reserved marinade.

Storage

Divide the pork and vegetables between six airtight containers or Ziploc bags; keep in your refrigerator for up to 3 to 5 days.

For freezing, place the pork and vegetables in airtight containers or heavy-duty freezer bags. Freeze for up to 4 months. Defrost in the refrigerator. Bon appétit!

Nutrition: 267 Calories; 10.6 g Fat; 5.3 g Carbs; 34.9 g Protein; 1.3 g Fiber

11 Pork Cutlets with Kale

Preparation Time: 2 hours (marinating time)

Cooking Time: 25 minutes

Servings: 6

Ingredients:

Sea salt and ground black pepper, to taste

2 tsp olive oil

¼ cup port wine

2 garlic cloves, smashed

2 tbsp oyster sauce

2 tbsp fresh lime juice

1 medium leek, sliced

2 bell peppers, chopped

2 cups kale

1½ lb pork cutlets

Directions:

Sprinkle the pork with salt and black pepper. Then, make the marinade by whisking one teaspoon of olive oil, wine, garlic, oyster sauce, and lime juice.

Let the pork marinate for about 2 hours in your refrigerator

Heat the remaining tsp of olive oil in a frying pan. Fry the leek and bell peppers for 4 to 5 minutes, stirring continuously until they have softened slightly; set aside.

In the same pan, sear the pork along with the marinade until browned on all sides.

Stir the reserved vegetables into the frying pan along with the kale. Continue to cook for 5 to 6 minutes more.

Storage

Place the pork chops and vegetables in airtight containers or Ziploc bags; keep in your refrigerator for 3 to 4 days.

Freeze the pork chops and vegetables in airtight containers or heavy-duty freezer bags. Freeze for up to 4 months. Defrost in the refrigerator. Bon appétit!

Nutrition: 234 Calories; 11 g Fat; 2 g Carbs; 29.8 g Protein; 0.9 g Fiber

Italian Keto Plate

Take your mind off of work for a bit and take your imagination to Italy with this amazing dish.

Preparation Time: 5 minutes

Cooking Time: 5 minutes

Servings: 1

Ingredients:

7 oz mozzarella cheese

7 oz fatty Italian deli meat

2 sliced tomatoes

⅓ cup olive oil

10 green or black olives

Salt and pepper to taste

Directions:

Put all of the ingredients on a plate or in your lunch tin. Serve with olive oil, and spice with salt & pepper to taste.

Nutrition: Carbohydrates: 24.7 g; Fat: 133 g; Protein: 108 g

13 Steak Tartare

You can have a themed lunch, almost every day with our cookbook. This wholesome Steak Tartare recipe will take you to France.

Preparation Time: 5 minutes

Cooking Time: 15 minutes

Servings: 2

Ingredients:

10 oz ground fatty beef cuts

2 tbsp capers

2 tbsp mild mustard

2 tbsp parmesan cheese

1 tbsp horseradish

2 separated eggs

1 cup baby lettuce

2 oz bottled chopped beetroot

Salt and pepper to taste

Directions:

Grate the horseradish and parmesan cheese. Wash and dry the lettuce, then arrange it on the plates.

Divide the ground, fatty beef into two equal parts. Form a patty and arrange it in the middle of the plate. Push an indentation in the middle of the patty with the back of a spoon.

Arrange the rest of the vegetables around the patty and on top of the lettuce.

Gently spoon the egg yolks on top of the patty. Season well with salt and pepper.

Nutrition: Carbohydrates: 7.2 g; Fat: 15.7 g; Protein: 50.1 g

14   Keto Deviled Eggs

Doesn't this recipe take you back to lazy weekends in the park, reading a book, and having a picnic?

Cooking Time: 10 minutes

Preparation Time: 5 minutes

Cooking Time: 10 minutes

Servings: 4

Ingredients:

4 hard-boiled eggs, shelled and halved

1 tsp Tabasco sauce

¼ cup full-fat mayo

8 cooked and peeled shrimp

Salt and pepper to taste

Directions:

Scoop out the yolk from the eggs and put the egg whites on a plate, with the hollowed sides pointing upwards.

In a bowl, mash the yolks. Then add Tabasco sauce, spices, and mayonnaise.

Spoon the mixture back into the hollowed egg whites and place a shrimp on top of the mixture.

Nutrition: Carbohydrates: 4.5 g; Fat: 10 g; Protein: 15.7 g

15 Oven-baked Brie Cheese

For the love of cheese! Who can disa-brie?

Cooking Time: 5 minutes

Preparation Time: 10 minutes

Cooking Time: 5 minutes

Servings: 1

Salmon Ingredients:

9 oz camembert or brie cheese wedge

1 peeled and crushed garlic clove

1 tbsp dried rosemary

2 oz pecan & walnuts mixed

1 tbsp extra virgin olive oil

Salt and pepper to taste

Directions:

Preheat the oven to 400°F.

Remove the wrapping from the cheese wedge. Place the whole cheese wedge on a baking sheet lined with foil or parchment paper.

Combine the remainder of the additives in a small mixing bowl, and mix well.

Place the mixture on top of the cheese wedge and place it in the oven.

Bake the cheese for a period of 10 minutes, remove out of the oven and serve immediately.

Nutrition: Carbohydrates: 12.4 g; Fat: 116.9 g; Protein: 56.9 g

Dinner Recipes

1 Keto Taco Cups

All the flavors of Mexico, in the palm of your hand, ready for you to enjoy.

Preparation Time: 10 minutes

Cooking Time: 20 minutes

Servings: 12

Ingredients:

2 cups grated parmesan cheese

1 tbsp olive oil

1 tbsp of garlic paste

1 small red onion, diced

1 lb ground (minced) fatty pork meat

1 tbsp smoked paprika spice

1 tbsp chili powder

1 tbsp cumin

Salt, pepper, and other aromatics, to taste

Tub of sour cream for serving

Chopped avocado, tomatoes, and coriander for serving

Directions:

Cut parchment paper (wax paper) into 12 squares of equal size. This will aid in transferring the cheese to the muffin tin.

Prepare a 12-inch regular muffin pan, and lightly coat with cooking spray or brush the edges of each individual tin with 2 tbsp of melted, unsalted butter.

Preheat the oven to 375°F, and line a baking sheet with the 12 prepared squares of parchment paper.

Place two tablespoons of parmesan cheese onto each individual piece of parchment paper. Ensure that the squares are about 2-3 inches apart.

Bake the cheese in the oven until the edges turn brown in color. Take out of the oven, and allow to cool for a few minutes.

Place a piece of baked cheese into each muffin tin, and use your hands to gently mold the cheese around the edges and the bottom of each tin cup.

In a sizable skillet, fire up the olive oil over medium heat. Add the onion and brown until soft. Next, add the garlic paste and minced pork meat. Cook the pork until it's not pink anymore.

Add the desired seasoning to the pan of meat. Place the baked cheese cups on a platter, and spoon the cooked meat into each cup.

Top with the avocado, coriander, tomato, and sour cream.

Nutrition: Carbohydrates: 1.6 g; Fat: 4.6 g; Protein: 12.7 g

2 Loaded Cauliflower Salad

All the crunch from the cauliflower florets and stuff with mouthfuls of cheese and fragrant, crunchy bacon bits.

Preparation Time: 10 minutes

Cooking Time: 30 minutes

Servings: 6

Ingredients:

1 large head of cauliflower, washed and cut into florets

¼ cup water

½ cup crispy bacon bits

½ sour cream

¼ full fat mayo

1 tbsp lemon juice

1½ grated cheddar cheese

¼ cup finely diced chives

Salt, pepper, and other aromatics, to taste

Directions:

Bring the water to a boil on the stove in a large pot or saucepan. Add the cauliflower florets to the pot, steam for 4 minutes. Drain the florets on a paper towel.

In a small frying pan, fry the bacon until crispy.

Combine the mayo, sour cream, and lemon juice in a large mixing bowl, and whisk well together. Add the cauliflower florets, and fold gently together.

Season well with the desired spices. Fold in the cheddar, chives, and bacon. Serve.

Nutrition: Carbohydrates: 13 g; Fat: 35 g; Protein: 19 g

3 Caprese Zoodles

Pasta can be healthy too when replacing the pasta with actual vegetable strips.

Preparation Time: 10 minutes

Cooking Time: 15 minutes

Servings: 4

Ingredients:

4 large, washed baby marrows (zucchini)

2 tbsp olive oil

2 cups cocktail tomatoes, cut lengthwise

1 cup mozzarella cheese balls

¼ cup basil leaves

2 tbsp red wine vinegar

Salt, pepper, and other aromatics, to taste

Directions:

Make zoodles from the baby marrow by turning and pushing it through a spiralizer tool.

In a large bowl, coat the fresh zoodles in olive oil, season well, and allow to marinate for 15 minutes. Add tomatoes, cheese, and basil, swirl gently until all of the additives are well-combined.

Dish the required amount on each serving plate. Drizzle with red wine vinegar. Serve.

Nutrition: Carbohydrates: 14.4 g; Fat: 9.5 g; Protein: 6 g

4 Keto Broccoli and Cheddar Soup

Some healthy vegetables, submerged in a luscious bath of cheddar cheese. Comfort at its best.

Preparation Time: 15 minutes

Cooking Time: 25 minutes

Servings: 6

Ingredients:

4 tbsp unsalted butter

1 large carrot, peeled and sliced into thin sticks

2 garlic cloves, peeled and crushed

¾ tbsp sweet, smoked paprika

¾ tbsp mustard powder

¾ tbsp onion powder

4 cups chicken stock or homemade chicken broth

6 cups small broccoli florets

6 oz plain cream cheese

4 cups shredded cheddar cheese

Salt, pepper, and other spices, to taste

Directions:

In a medium-sized skillet, melt the unsalted butter. Then add the carrot and garlic, and cook until the garlic is fragrant. Normally, this takes about 3 minutes.

Next, combine the paprika, mustard, cayenne, and onion powder, and stir well. Add the chicken stock or broth to the mix, and season well.

Add the broccoli florets to the mix and cook for 5 minutes, until tender. Combine the cheddar and cream cheese, and stir continuously until the cheese has melted.

Season if needed, and serve warm.

Nutrition: Carbohydrates: 10.1 g; Fat: 43.5 g; Protein: 24.9 g

5 Egg Roll Bowls

This eating plan is so good to you, that you are even permitted to have your favorite egg rolls. Unleash the flavor!

Preparation Time: 10 minutes

Cooking Time: 25 minutes

Servings: 4

Ingredients:

1 tbsp avocado oil

1 garlic clove, peeled and crushed

1 tbsp ginger

1 lb. ground pork

1 tbsp sesame oil

½ red onion, finely diced

1 cup grated carrot

¼ head of green cabbage, thinly shredded

½ cup low-sodium soy sauce

1 tbsp sriracha paste

1 scallion, finely chopped

1 tbsp mixed seeds (sunflower, poppy, sesame)

Salt, pepper, and other spices, as desired.

Directions:

In a sizable skillet, heat the avocado oil, over medium heat. Add the garlic and ginger to the skillet and cook for 3 minutes, until fragrant. Add the ground pork, cook until the meat no longer has any pink hues.

Move the pork to the one side of the pan. Add the sesame oil, onion, carrot, and cabbage to the same pan. Stir and combine this with the meat. Combine the sriracha paste and soy sauce.

Cook for 6-7 minutes, until the cabbage is tender. Transfer to dishes for serving and season to taste. Top with mixed seeds, and scallion.

Nutrition:

Carbohydrates: 11 g; Fat: 32 g; Protein: 22 g

6 Quesadillas - Keto Style

This eating plan is so good to you, that you are even permitted to have your favorite egg rolls. Unleash the flavor!

Preparation Time: 10 minutes

Cooking Time: 25 minutes

Servings: 4

Ingredients:

1 tbsp olive oil

1 bell pepper, diced

⅓ red onion, finely diced

½ tsp chili powder

3 cups parmesan cheese, grated

3 cups smoked chicken, shredded

1 avocado, peeled and thinly diced

1 scallion, finely chopped

3 cups sharp cheddar, grated

Salt, pepper, and other spices, to taste

Tub of sour cream for serving

Directions:

Line two baking sheets with parchment paper (wax paper) and preheat the oven to 400°F.

Heat the olive oil in a medium-sized frying pan. Combine the pepper, red onion, and season well. Cook for 5 minutes until soft, remove from heat, and add to a plate.

In a mixing bowl, combine the cheddar cheese and parmesan cheeses. Scoop 1½ cups of the cheese mixture onto the middle of each lined baking sheet. With a spoon, spread it out into a layer and shape to simulate a flour tortilla.

Transfer to the oven and bake the cheese until the edges turn crispy, and the cheese is melted. Remove from the oven. Add the pepper and onion mixture, chicken, and slices of avocado on one side of each of the tortillas.

Allow to cool for a few minutes, and fold over the side that does not have the filling, into a folded omelet. Return to the oven for 4 minutes. Repeat the process with the leftover cheese.

Cut the quesadilla into quarters, serve with sour cream and scallion.

Nutrition: Carbohydrates: 12.8 g; Fat: 46.7 g; Protein: 99.9 g

7 Cheeseburger Tomatoes

No one really eats both the buns right? Now you eat your cheeseburger completely guilt-free.

Preparation Time: 5 minutes

Cooking Time: 20 minutes

Servings: 4

Ingredients:

1 tbsp olive oil

1 medium-sized red onion, diced

2 garlic cloves, peeled and crushed

1 lb ground beef (not lean)

1 tbsp ketchup. Check for a brand that does not have added sugar

1 tbsp keto-friendly mustard

4 medium-sized tomatoes

⅔ cup sharp cheddar, grated

¼ cup spinach, shredded

½ tsp chili powder

4 slices of pickle

Salt, pepper, and other spices, as desired.

Directions:

Fire up the olive oil in a medium-sized skillet over medium heat. Put in the onion, and fry until softened. Join the garlic, and cook for 3 minutes. Add the beef, and cook until the meat is no longer pink. Break the big chunks of beef by breaking it up with a spoon.

Drain the remaining grease in the pan. Season with desired spices. Add ketchup and mustard and stir well.

Wash and dry the tomatoes, and bring them to stand on their stem sides. Cut the tomatoes into 6 equal wedges, but don't cut it all the way through. Gently open the wedges and spoon the beef mixture equally into the 4 tomatoes. Add a slice of pickle on top.

Nutrition: Carbohydrates: 15.4 g; Fat: 20 g; Protein: 37.1 g

8 Three Cheese Chicken and Cauliflower

Another great alternative to pasta that tastes even better than the original dish.

Preparation Time: 40 minutes

Cooking Time: 1 hour

Servings: 8

Filling Ingredients:

1 tbsp olive oil

1 leek, thinly diced

2 cups ground chicken

1 pt. button mushrooms, washed and sliced

1 packet baby spinach, washed and shredded

1 cup cream cheese

1 tsp tarragon

½ canned tomato paste

1 cup mozzarella cheese, grated

Salt, pepper, and other spices, to taste

Lasagna Sheet Ingredients:

1 large cauliflower head

½ cup parmesan cheese

2 whole eggs

Non-stick spray

Directions:

Heat up the oven to 356°F prior to starting out.

Chop up half of the cauliflower head, and add to a blender or food processor. Chop finely. This can also be done manually by hand, using a sharp knife and cutting board. Move the chopped cauliflower and place it aside in a mixing bowl. Repeat the process with the other half.

Add 2 cups of water. Cover the bowl with cling wrap or a lid, and microwave on a high setting until it's tender, stirring occasionally throughout the cooking process. Once done, drain the excess liquid through a sieve. Return to the bowl and add the parmesan cheese, egg, and season well. Combine the mixture.

Using two baking trays, line them with parchment paper. Divide the mixture equally between the two baking sheets. Use your fingers to press the mixture into the baking sheets in rectangles along the edges. Put in the oven and cook until the mixture has dried out. Take out of the oven and allow to cool. Cut into a width of 10 cm to make lasagna sheets.

Heat the olive oil in a large skillet over high heat. Add the leek, and reduce the heat to low. Cook until soft. Add the chicken, and break the lumps of meat into smaller pieces with a wooden spoon. Cook for at least 5 minutes. Add the mushrooms, and cook for 5 minutes.

Next, add the spinach, and cook until wilted. Add the cream cheese and cook until melted. Stir in the tarragon, and season according to taste.

Coat an oven-proof baking dish with the cooking spray (24-cm top measurement and 19-cm base measurement). Brush the base and the edges of the baking dish with the tomato paste. Place 2 sheets over the tomato paste.

Scoop ½ of the chicken mixture on top and sprinkle with ⅓ cup of mozzarella cheese. Add another layer of cauliflower and repeat the process. End with the remaining tomato paste and mozzarella on top. Bake for 30 minutes in the oven. Take out and allow to rest outside the oven for 7 minutes until firm.

Nutrition: Carbohydrates: 16.1 g; Fat: 19.5 g; Protein: 23. 5 g

9 Garlic Butter Salmon with Lemon Asparagus Skillet

One of the great advantages of this dish is that it is packed with flavor, and can be cooked in one pan. It's one of the quickest dishes to prepare in our cookbook.

Preparation Time: 5 minutes

Cooking Time: 25 minutes

Servings: 2

Filling Ingredients:

1 medium salmon, divided into 4 equal portions

2 bundles of green asparagus, washed and trimmed

1 tbsp extra virgin olive oil

2 tbsp garlic flakes

½ cup dry white wine

110 g of unsalted butter

1 tbsp sriracha sauce

3 oz lemon juice

1 tbsp coriander

1 tbsp parsley

4 lemon cheeks for garnish and drizzle afterward

Salt, pepper, and other spices, to taste

Directions:

Pat the salmon chunks dry on both sides with a kitchen towel, and place them on a cutting board. Season well with desired spices, and rub the spices across the surface of the salmon. Marinate in the salt rub.

In a medium pan, add the asparagus, and add water, until the vegetables are covered, and cook for 2 minutes. Transfer to an ice-water bath immediately after the 3 minutes have elapsed.

Heat the olive oil in a non-stick cast-iron skillet over medium heat. Sear the salmon on both sides. Gently flip it over with a spatula each time, so as not to disturb the flaky texture of the fish. Once the salmon is golden brown on both sides, remove from the skillet and transfer to a plate.

In the skillet that the fish was cooked, add the minced garlic and cook for 3 minutes until fragrant. Add the white wine, and reduce the heat to cook the alcohol away. Add the butter, lemon juice, sriracha paste, and parsley. Stir to combine.

Add the asparagus to the pan, and cook for 2 minutes. Add the salmon back into the pan, and reheat. Gently turning the chunks over.

Sprinkle with parsley and add the cheeks of lemon. Serve immediately.

Nutrition: Carbohydrates: 13.51 g; Fat: 38.57 g; Protein: 42.09 g

Hearty Shrimp Curry

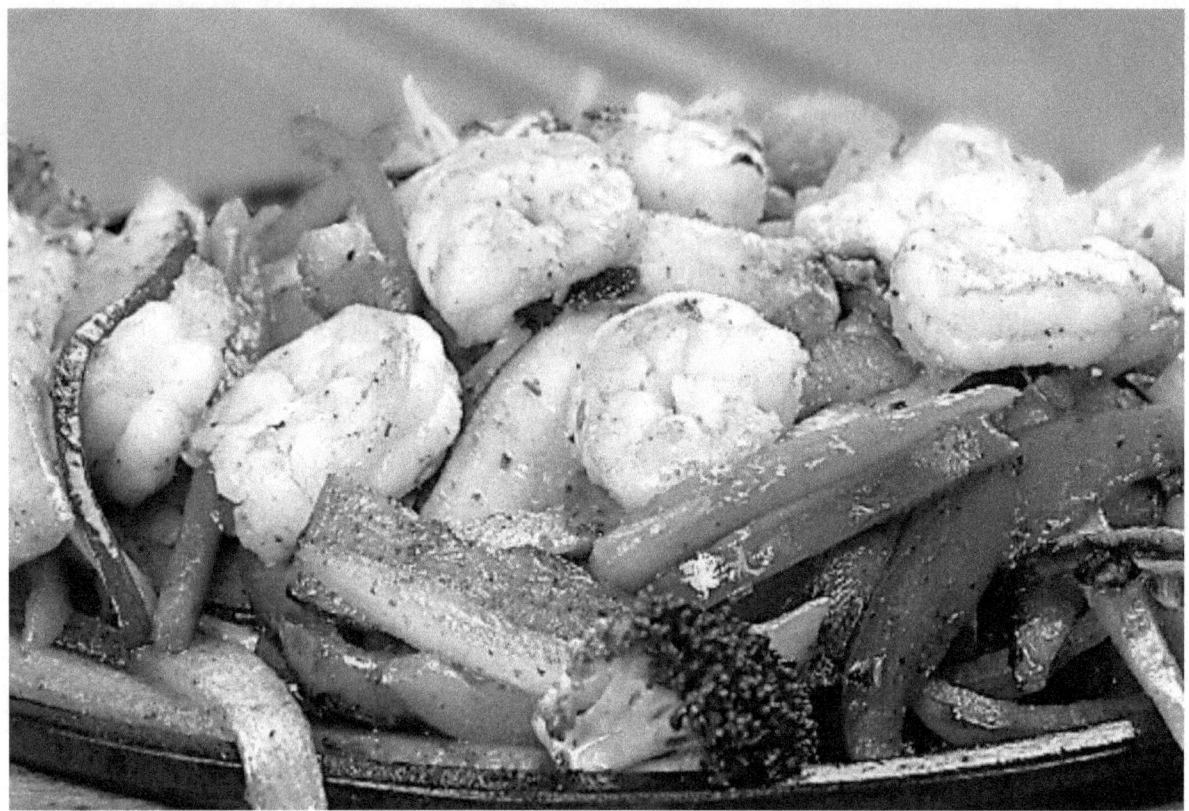

Preparation Time: 5 minutes

Cooking Time: 10 minutes

Servings: 2

Ingredients:

2 tbsp Green Curry paste

1 cup vegetable stock

1 cup coconut milk

6 oz pre-cooked shrimp

5 oz Broccoli florets

3 tbsp chopped cilantro

2 tbsp coconut oil

1 tbsp soy sauce

Juice of half of a lime

1 medium-sized spring onion, chopped

1 tsp crushed roasted garlic

1 tsp minced garlic

1 tsp fish sauce

½ tsp turmeric

¼ tsp Xanthan gum

½ cup sour cream

Directions:

Place a pan over medium heat and add two tablespoons of coconut oil.

Add minced ginger, chopped up onion and cook for a minute.

Add turmeric and curry paste.

Add the soy sauce and fish sauce, and mix.

Add a cup of vegetable stock and a cup of coconut milk.

Stir well and add green curry paste. Simmer.

Add ¼ tsp of Xanthan gum and mix well.

After a while, you will notice that the curry will begin to thicken, that will be the moment when you are going to be needing to add the florets and stir them finely.

Add the fresh chopped cilantro.

Once you have a nice consistency, add the weighed, pre-cooked shrimp and lime juice.

Allow the mix to simmer for a few minutes and season with pepper and salt.

Serve with sour cream.

Enjoy!

Nutrition: Protein: 27 g; Carbs: 8.9 g; Fats: 31 g; Calories: 454

11 Ancient Salmon Glaze and Teriyaki

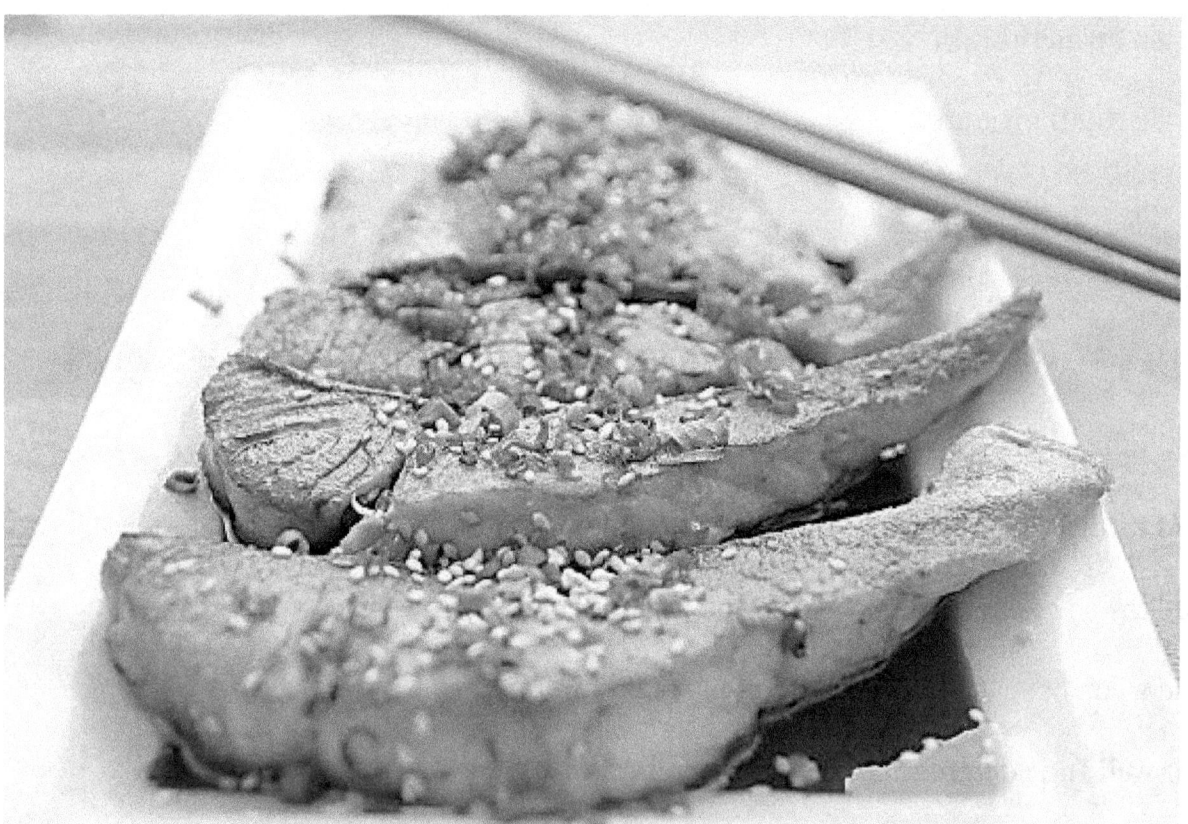

Preparation Time: 10 minutes

Cooking Time: 10 minutes

Servings: 2

Ingredients:

10 oz of salmon fillet

2 tbsp soy sauce

2 tsp sesame oil

1 tbsp rice vinegar

1 tsp minced ginger

2 tsp minced garlic

1 tbsp red boat fish sauce

1 tbsp sugar-free ketchup

2 tbsp dry white wine

Directions:

Toss in all of the ingredients in a small-sized bowl. Just make sure not to toss the sesame oil, white wine, and ketchup.

Marinate for about 10-15 minutes.

Bring down the pan to a nice heat and toss in the sesame oil.

Once the smoke is seen, toss the fish with the skin side down.

Let it cook until crispy.

Flip it and cook the other side. Each side should take about 3-4 minutes.

Pour in the marinade into the fish and let it boil.

Slowly remove the fish from the pan and pour in the ketchup alongside the white wine to the liquid in the pan.

Simmer for 5 minutes and serve as a side.

Nutrition: Protein: 33 g; Carbs: 2.5 g; Fats: 23.5 g; Calories: 370

12   Extremely Low Carb Chicken Satay

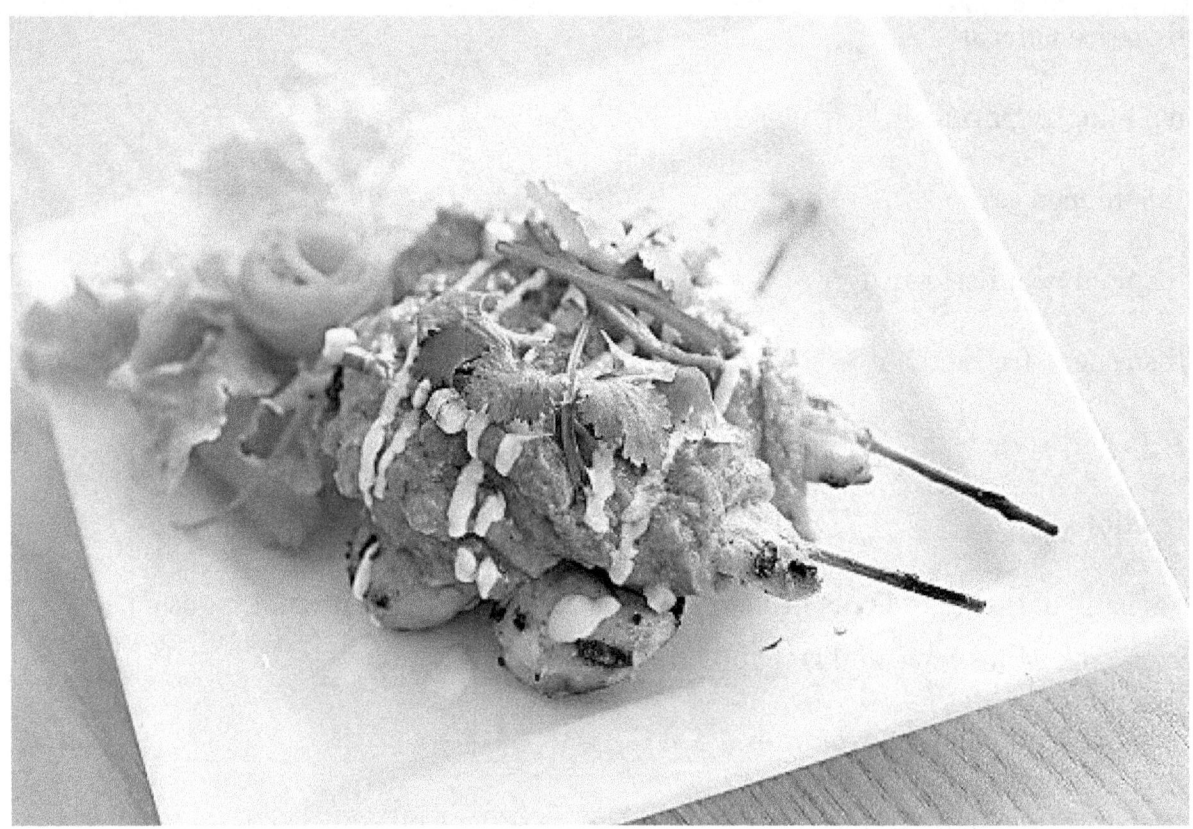

Preparation Time: 5 minutes

Cooking Time: 5 minutes

Servings: 1

Ingredients:

1 lb ground chicken

4 tbsp soy sauce

2 onion springs

1/3 of a yellow pepper

1 tbsp erythritol

1 tbsp rice vinegar

2 tsp sesame oil

2 tsp chili paste

1 tsp minced garlic

1/3 tsp cayenne pepper

¼ tsp paprika

Juice of half a lime

Directions:

Add 2 teaspoons of sesame oil to a pan and heat it over medium-high heat.

Add ground chicken to your pan and allow it to brown.

Add the rest of the ingredients and mix well.

Once the mixture has reached your desired texture, add the spring onions and sliced yellow pepper.

Mix and serve!

Nutrition: Protein: 105 g; Carbs: 18 g; Fats: 69 g; Calories: 1180

13   Spicy Hot Chicken and Pepper Soup

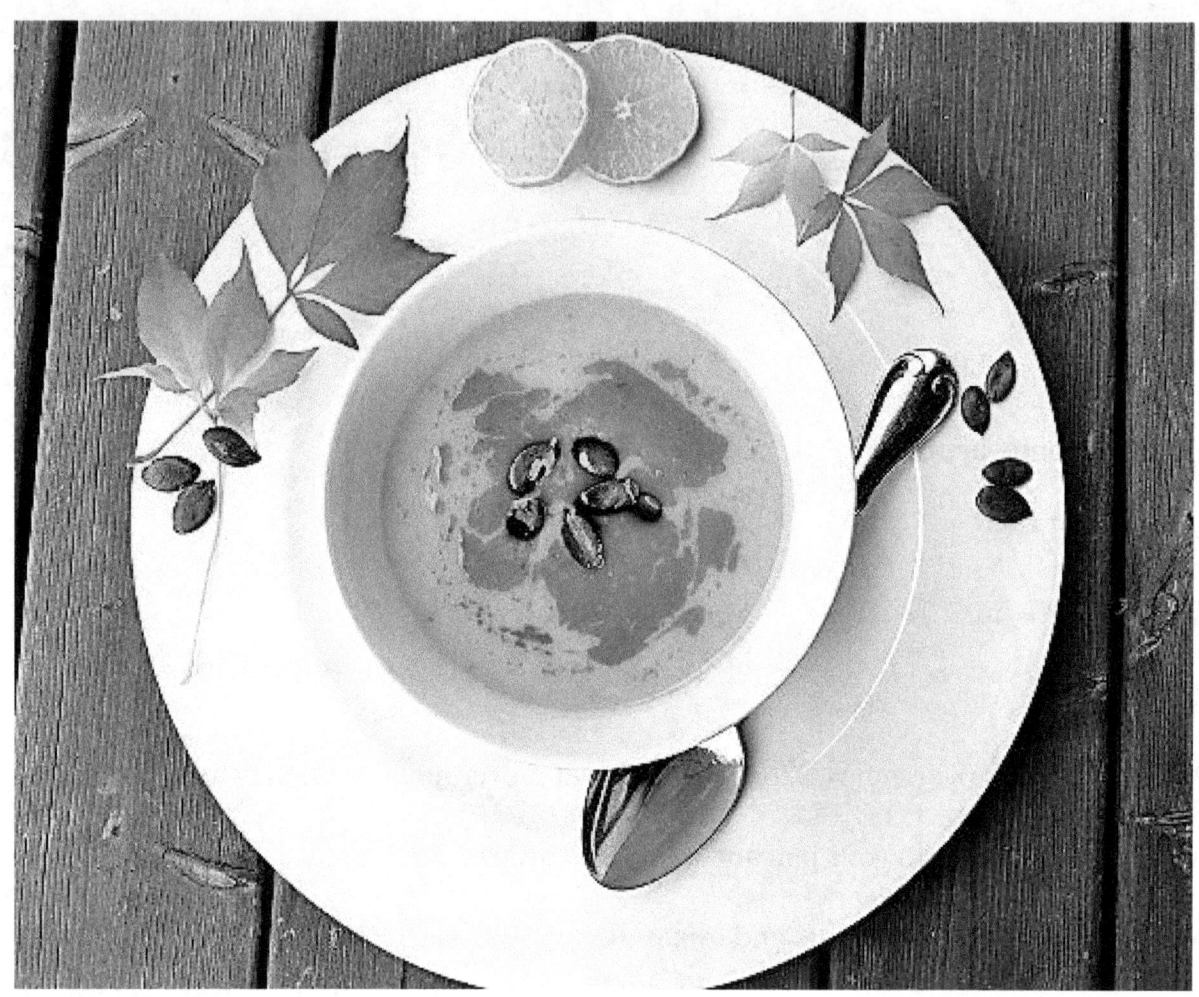

Preparation Time: 5 minutes

Cooking Time: 10 minutes

Servings: 5

Ingredients:

1 tsp coriander seeds

2 tbsp olive oil

2 sliced chili pepper

2 cups chicken broth

2 cups water

1 tsp turmeric

½ tsp ground cumin

4 tbsp tomato paste

16 oz chicken thigh

2 tbsp butter

1 medium-sized avocado

2 oz Queso Fresco

4 tbsp chopped cilantro

Juice of a half lime

Salt and pepper as required

Directions:

Cut the chicken thigh into small portions.

Take a pan and place it over medium heat. Add oil and allow it to heat up.

Add chicken pieces and brown them on both sides. Transfer to a platter and keep it on the side.

Add olive oil to the pan and add coriander seeds. Toast until fragrant.

Pour water and broth, and simmer over low heat.

Season with pepper, turmeric, salt, and ground cumin.

Bring the mix to a simmer. Add tomato paste, butter, and stir well.

Simmer for 10 minutes and add the lime juice.

Add the cooked chicken thigh and mix well.

Garnish with avocado, cilantro, and Queso Fresco.

Enjoy!

Nutrition: Protein: 28 g; Carbs: 10.8 g; Fats: 27 g; Calories: 395

14   Butter Fried Kale and Pork With Cranberries

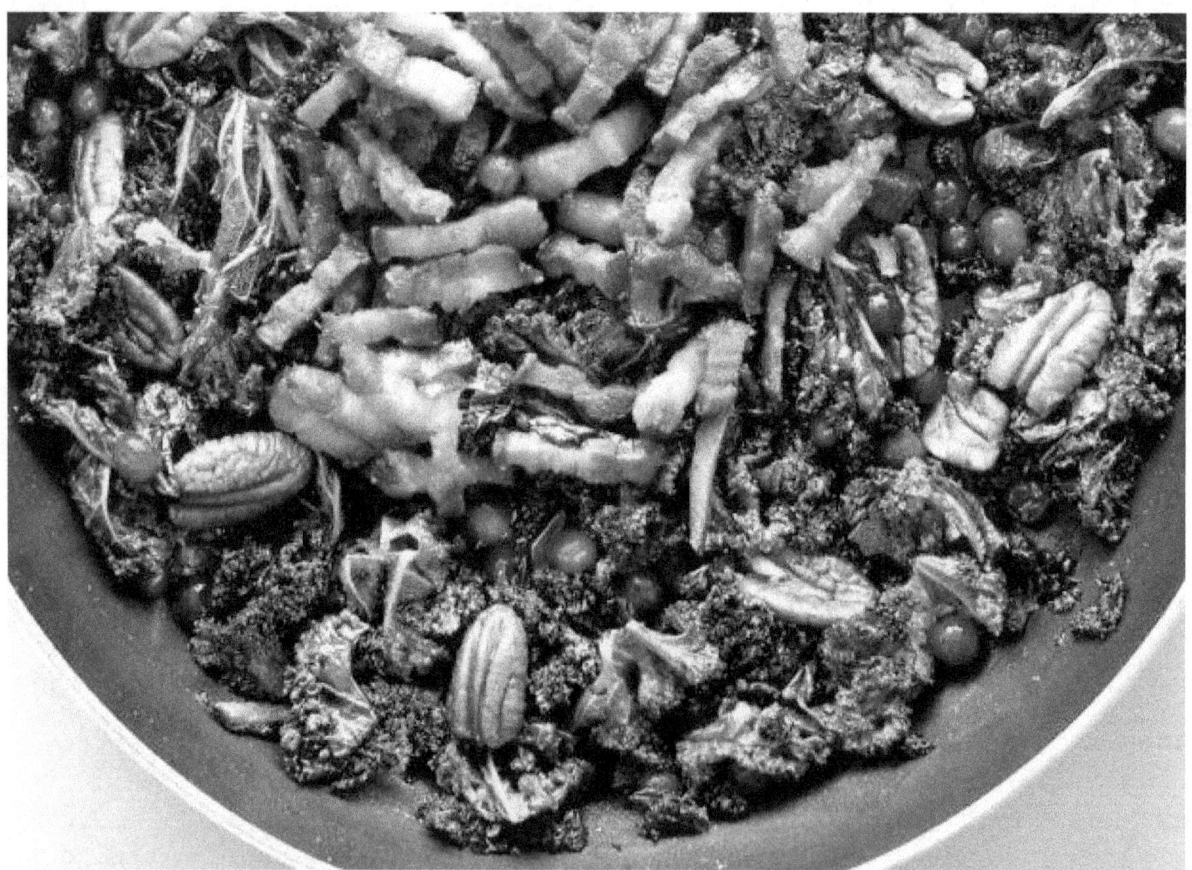

Preparation Time: 10 minutes

Cooking Time: 10 minutes

Servings: 4

Ingredients:

3 oz butter

1 lb kale

¾ lb smoked pork belly

2 oz pecans

½ cup frozen cranberries

Directions:

Rinse, trim and chop your kale into large-sized chunks. Keep it on the side.

Cut the pork belly into strips and fry them in butter over medium-high heat.

Once they are golden brown and crispy, add kale to the pan and fry for a few minutes.

Remove the heat and add cranberries and nuts to the pan.

Stir well and serve!

Nutrition: Protein: 21 g; Carbs: 10 g; Fats: 12 g; Calories: 223

Amazing Keto Zucchini Hash

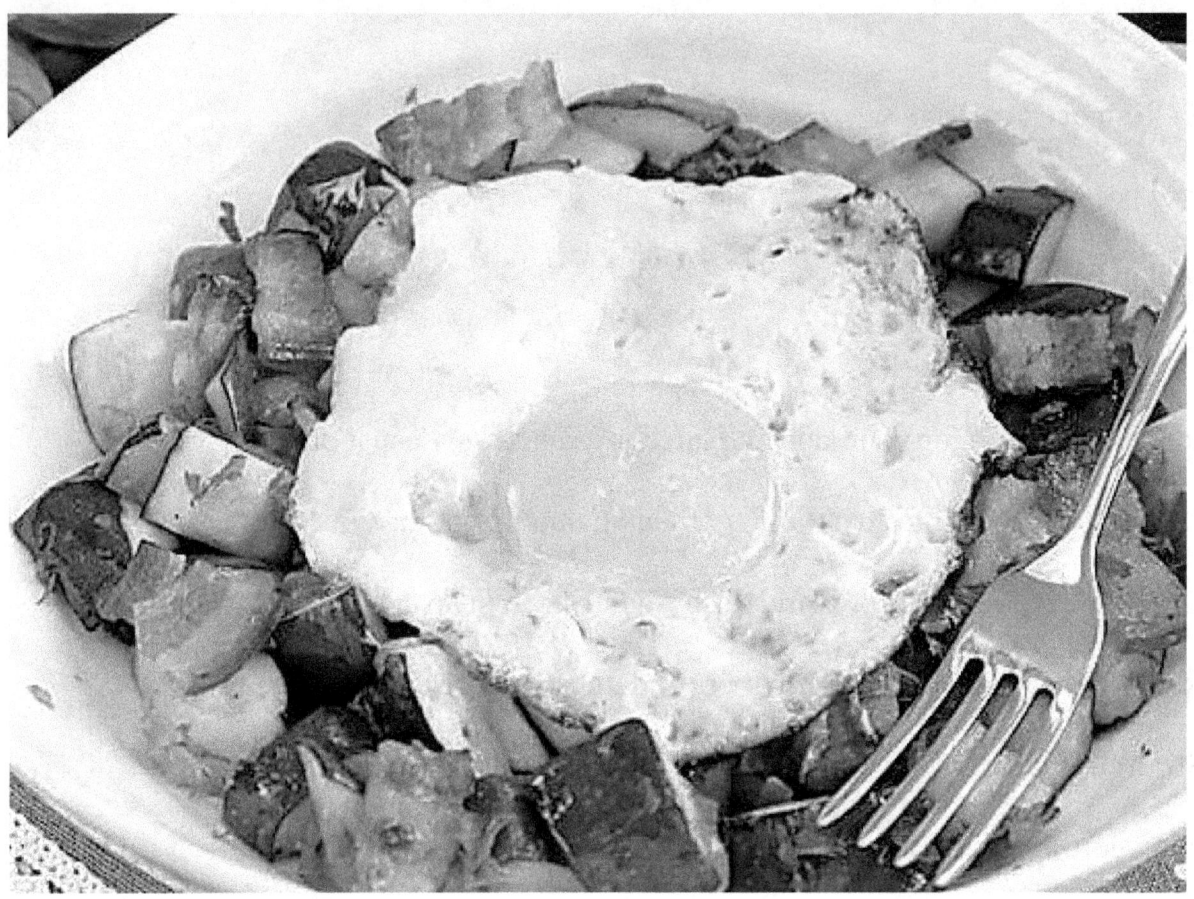

Preparation Time: 10 minutes

Cooking Time: 10-15 minutes

Servings: 4

Ingredients:

1 medium-sized zucchini

2 slices of bacon

½ of a small white onion

1 tbsp coconut oil

1 tbsp freshly chopped parsley

¼ tsp salt

1 large egg

Directions:

Peel and finely chop the onion. Slice the bacon.

Sweat the onions over medium heat and add the bacon. Make sure to stir from time to time to ensure that they are lightly browned.

Dice the zucchini into medium pieces.

Add zucchini to your pan and cook for 10-15 minutes. Remove the heat and add chopped parsley.

Top with a fried egg and enjoy!

Nutrition: Protein: 17 g; Carbs: 6 g; Fats: 35 g; Calories: 423

Poultry Recipes

1 Espetada

Espetada is a traditional dish in Portuguese cuisine that originated in Portugal. It is the technique of making food on skewers, and they are cooked over hot coals or wood chips. However, you can also bake the Espetadas in the oven. They turn out just as delicious.

Preparation Time: 10 minutes + 60 minutes (minimum) marinating time

Cooking Time: 30 minutes

Servings: 4

Ingredients:

8 chicken pieces (drumstick and thighs)

1 cup full cream yogurt

1 tsp Dijon mustard

4 tbsp fresh ginger (grated)

4 tbsp crushed garlic

1 tsp chili flakes (optional)

1 tsp garam masala

½ tsp salt

Ingredients:

You can either make the Espetadas in the oven or barbeque them. If baking them in the oven, preheat the oven to 350°F (180°C).

In a medium-size bowl mix the yogurt, Dijon mustard, ginger, garlic, chili flakes, garam masala, and Himalayan salt.

Place the chicken into the mixture and make sure it covers all of the chicken.

Cover the bowl with cling wrap and place in the refrigerator for at least 1 hour. For best results, place overnight.

If you are using wooden skewers, then soak them in hot water for at least an hour.

Thread the marinated chicken onto the skewers (A thigh and a drumstick on one skewer).

Place the Espetadas into an ovenproof pan and bake for 30 minutes or until done. If barbequing, place the chicken skewers onto the hot grill. Use tongs to turn the skewers occasionally until slightly charred and cooked through, about 20-30 minutes.

Quick Tip: If the juices run clear, the chicken is fully cooked. If the fluid has a slight pink tinge to it, it needs more cooking time.

Nutrition: Fat: 17.3 g; Protein: 31.4 g; Carbs: 7.6 g; Fiber: 0.8 g; Calories: 316

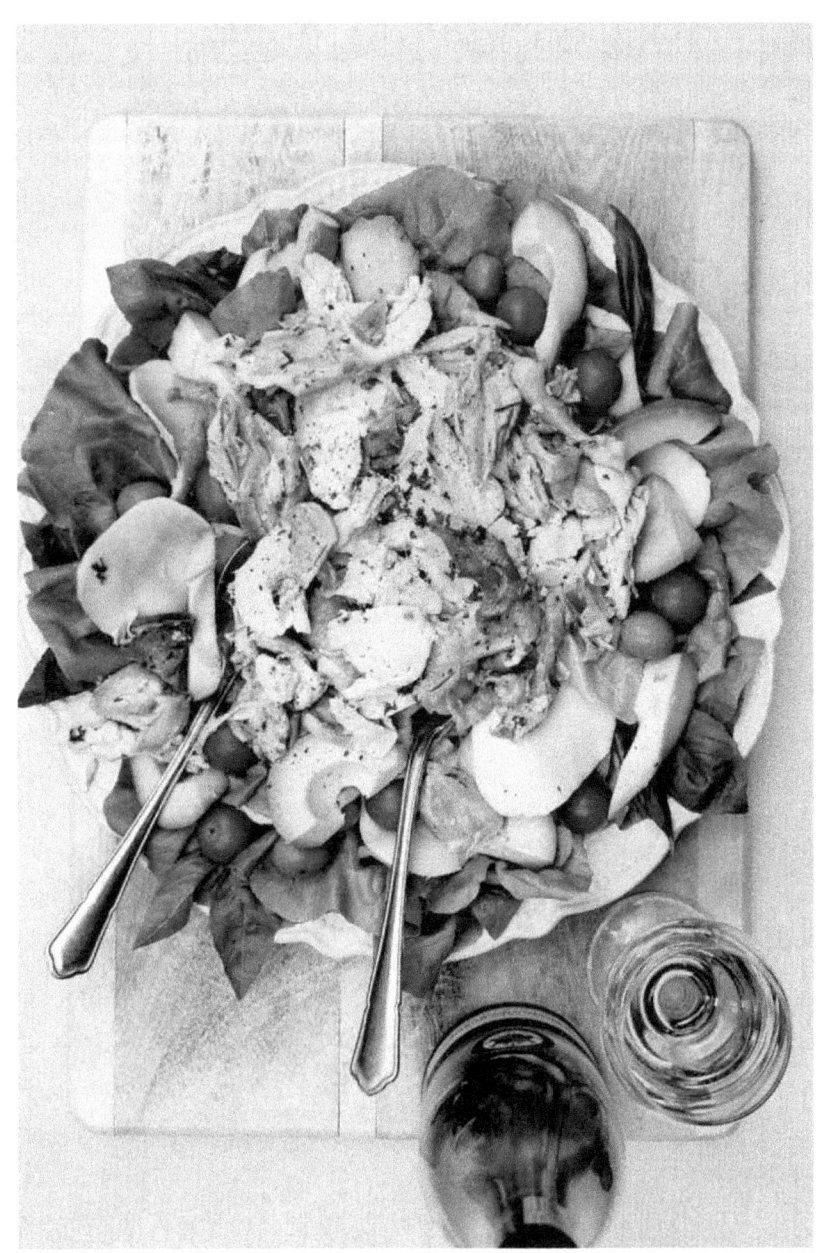

2 Chicken Caprese Salad with Avocado

Preparation Time: 15 minutes

Cooking Time: 20 minutes

Servings: 2

Ingredients:

Olive Oil and Balsamic Vinegar Marinade and Salad Dressing

⅓ cup balsamic vinegar

2 cloves crushed garlic

⅛ tsp black pepper (add more to taste)

½ tsp salt (add more to taste)

1 tbsp Dijon mustard

⅔ cup olive oil

Caprese Salad

2 chicken fillets with skin

1 tbsp butter

2 cups shredded lettuce leaves

½ avocado, sliced

½ cup cherry or Roma tomatoes

½ cup mozzarella (sliced)

1/3 cup basil leaves

Salt and pepper, to taste

Directions:

Start with the marinade/salad dressing first.

Take a medium-sized bowl and mix the balsamic vinegar, garlic, black pepper, salt, Dijon mustard, and olive oil. Taste and add more salt and pepper if necessary.

Take about half of the marinade and put it into a bowl with the chicken. Make sure that all the chicken pieces are covered in the marinade. Marinate for at least 30 minutes.

While the chicken marinates, get started with the salad.

Take a flat salad bowl and arrange the lettuce, avocados, tomatoes, mozzarella, and basil to your liking.

Melt the butter in a medium-sized pan and fry the marinated chicken fillets for about a total of 7 minutes on each side, turning every few minutes until done. Let the chicken rest for about 3 minutes and slice it up (if you prefer your chicken to be cold in the salad, let it cool down completely, then cut it into slices).

Place the chicken on top of the salad and drizzle on the salad dressing.

Quick Tip:

If you want to know whether an avocado is ripe, simply peel back the small stem or cap at the top of the avocado. If it comes away easily and you find green underneath, you've got the perfect avocado that's ripe and ready to eat.

Nutrition: Fat: 70 g; Protein: 68 g; Carbs: 15.6 g; Fiber: 5.1 g; Calories: 967

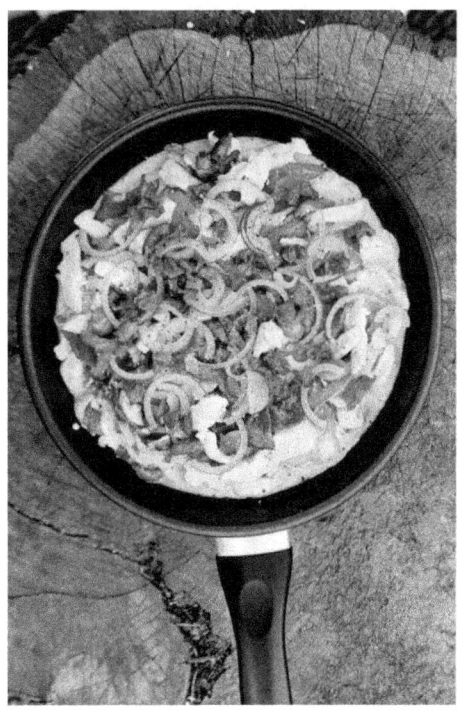

3 Creamy Chicken with Salami and Olives

Preparation Time: 5 minutes

Cooking Time: 30 minutes

Servings: 2

Ingredients:

2 chicken breasts cut into strips. Remove the skin and set aside.

½ onion sliced

½ red bell pepper sliced

1 tsp crushed garlic

10 salami slices cut in quarters (sugar-free)

3 tbsp butter

1 cup chicken stock

½ cup green olives

1 cup cream

Salt and pepper to taste

Method:

In a large pan, melt the butter over medium heat.

Add the onion, bell pepper, garlic, salami, and chicken skin. Fry until soft and slightly brown.

Add the stock and olives, and reduce by half.

Add the cream and reduce by a third.

Add the chicken pieces and cook until the chicken is cooked.

Season with salt and pepper to taste.

Quick Tip: Letting the salami get to room temperature makes it easier to cut and brings out the best salami flavor. Always check your ingredients to ensure there are no hidden carbs.

Nutrition: Fat: 102.7 g; Protein: 49.8 g; Carbs: 8 g; Fiber: 4.1 g; Calories: 1167

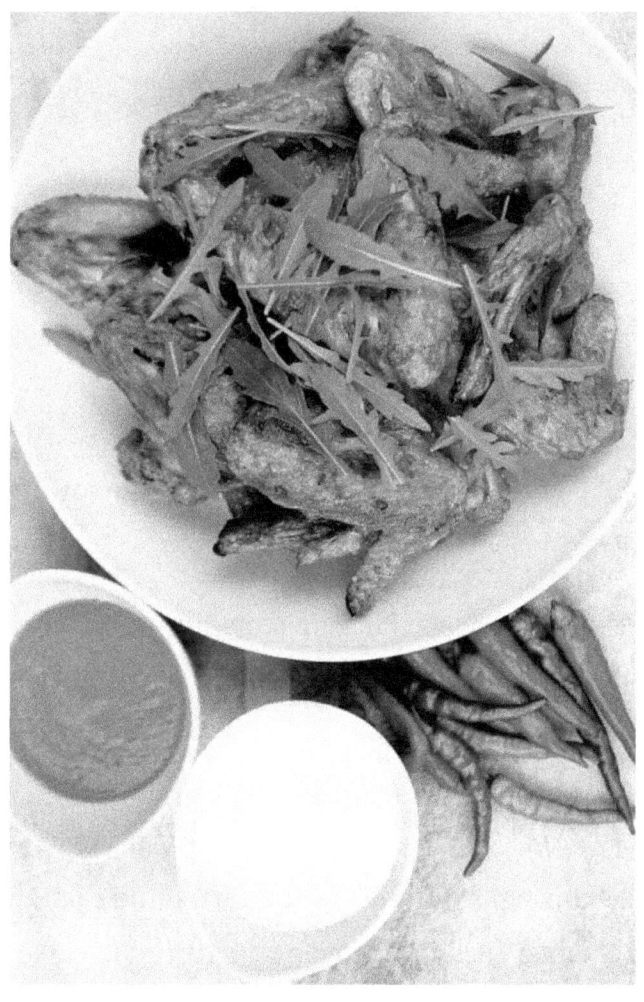

4 Buffalo Wings, Hot Sauce & Blue Cheese Dip

Preparation Time: 15 minutes

Cooking Time: 70 minutes

Servings: 4

Ingredients:

2 lb/1kg chicken wings

2½ tsp baking powder

½ tsp salt

Hot Sauce

Blue Cheese Dip

Directions:

Preheat the oven to 250°F (120°C). Put one oven shelf in the lower quarter of the oven and one in the top quarter.

Pat the chicken dry with paper towels. Place in a medium-size bowl and sprinkle the baking powder and salt over it. Toss well so that the chicken is evenly coated.

Line a tray with foil and place a baking rack on top of it. Place the chicken on the baking rack and place it in the lower quarter of the oven. Bake for 30 minutes.

When done, remove the chicken from the lower quarter and turn the oven up to 425°F/220°C. Put the chicken back in the oven (the top quarter) and bake for another 40 to 50 minutes.

The chicken is done when the skin is nice and crispy. Drizzle over some hot sauce and serve with the blue cheese dip.

Quick Tip: The trick to getting your chicken wings ultra-crispy is using baking powder. How exactly does adding baking powder make the wings crispy? When adding the baking powder, the pH level on the skin rises, and this causes the peptide bonds to break down. Now your chicken will be ultra-crispy and golden brown.

Nutrition (Baked Wings): Fat: 48 g; Protein: 67 g; Carbs: 0.7 g; Fiber: 0 g; Calories: 722

Nutrition (Baked Wings with Red Hot Sauce): Fat: 60 g; Protein: 68 g; Carbs: 3.3 g; Fiber: 0.4 g; Calories: 843

Nutrition (Blue Cheese Dip): Fat: 16 g; Protein: 2.78 g; Carbs: 2.4 g; Fiber: 0.2 g; Calories: 155

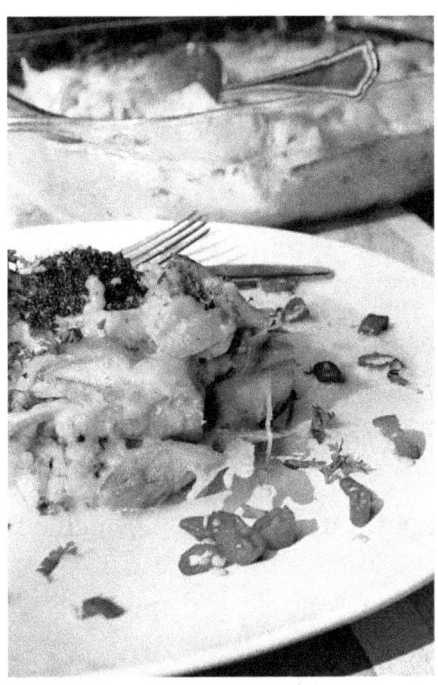

5 Tacos

Preparation Time: 10 minutes

Cooking Time: 25 minutes

Servings: 2

Ingredients:

Taco shells (makes 2 taco shells)

120 g shredded cheddar cheese

Chicken:

Grilled Chicken Breast Page

Filling:

½ cup mashed avocado

½ cup chopped tomatoes

¼ cup chopped onions

¼ cup sour cream

Parsley to garnish (optional)

Salt and pepper to taste

Directions:

Taco Shells:

Preheat the oven to 375°F (190°C)

Line a pan with parchment paper. I like to trace 2.5-inch circles on each parchment.

Measure 30 g of shredded cheese per circle and spread evenly.

Bake for 5 minutes or until little holes have appeared on the surface, and the edges begin to brown.

Remove from the oven and let cool for just a second. Remove to wooden spoons or spatulas suspended by glasses to shape taco shells.

Cool completely.

Chicken:

Cut the chicken into small pieces.

Take the tacos and add the fillings –first the chicken, then the avocado, tomatoes, onions, and sour cream. Garnish with some fresh herb such as parsley.

Season with salt and pepper to taste.

Quick Tip: While you are busy making these tacos, make a few extra because they freeze quite well and will save you some time when you make a taco dish again.

Nutrition: Fat: 63 g; Protein: 76 g; Carbs: 11.5 g; Fiber: 5 g; Calories: 918

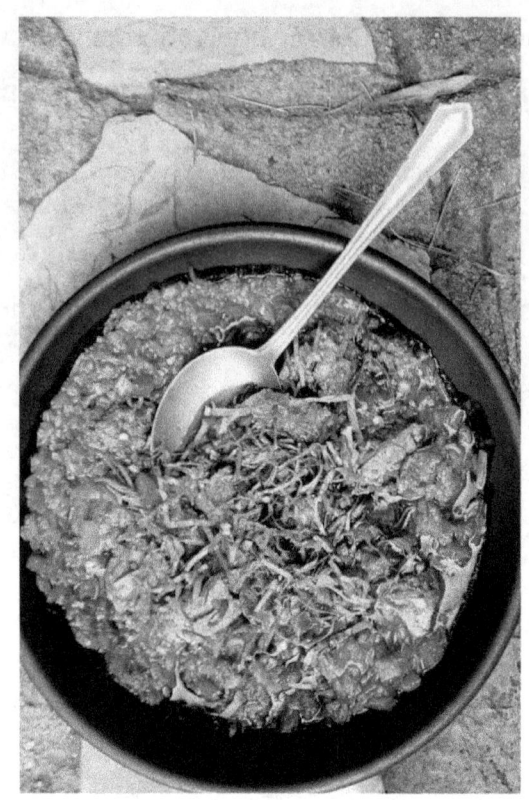

6 Chicken Livers

Preparation Time: 10 minutes

Cooking Time: 25 minutes

Servings: 2

Ingredients:

250 g chicken livers

4tbsp butter

½ large onion finely chopped

3 cloves of garlic, crushed

2 red chilies, finely chopped (optional)

½ cup white wine

1 tbsp tomato paste

1 tbsp lemon juice

1 tbsp olive oil

Salt and pepper

½ cup basil, finely chopped

Directions:

For the sauce

Place a medium-size frying pan on medium heat. Add 2 tablespoons of butter and the onion. Sauté until soft. Now add the garlic and chili. Sauté until fragrant.

Add the wine and reduce by half. Add the tomato paste and lemon juice, and let it simmer for one minute. Set aside.

Take a heavy-based frying pan and add remaining butter and olive oil. Add the chicken livers and fry them till they are beautiful and brown on both sides.

Add the sauce to the chicken livers and let it simmer until the livers are cooked.

Season to taste with salt and pepper. Now garnish with the fresh basil, and you are ready to serve.

Quick Tip: To clean your chicken livers, place the livers in cold water and let them soak for 15 minutes. This gives the water time to clot the blood, which will make it easier to remove. Drain the water and pat the livers dry with a paper towel. Look for connective tissue and trim it from the meat. Chop the liver in even, bite-size pieces.

Nutrition: Fat: 36 g; Protein: 22.6g; Carbs: 7.8 g; Fiber: 1.2 g; Calories: 489

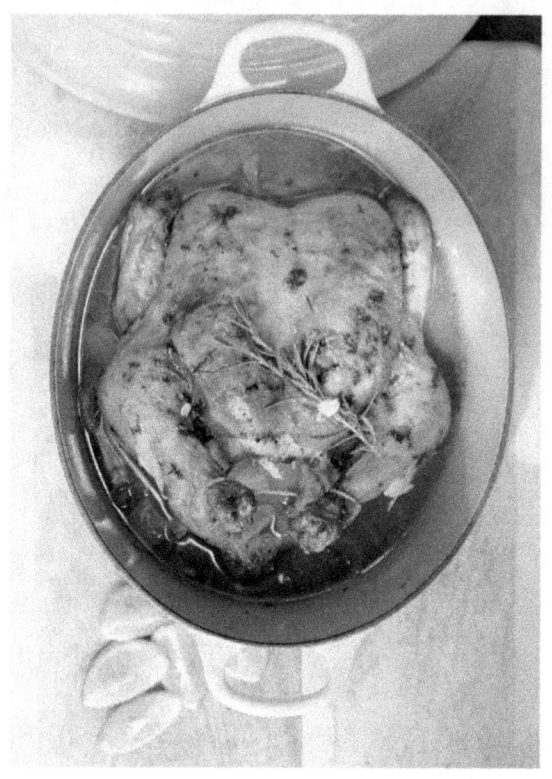

7 Chicken And Herb Butter With Keto Zucchini Roll-Ups

Preparation Time: 15 minutes

Cooking Time: 40 minutes

Servings: 4

Ingredients:

zucchini roll-ups:

1½ lb (680 g) zucchini

½ tsp salt

3 oz (85 g) butter

6 oz (170 g) mushrooms, finely chopped

6 oz (170 g) cream cheese

6 oz (170 g) shredded cheddar cheese

½ green bell pepper, chopped

2 oz (57 g) air-dried chorizo, chopped

1 egg

1 tsp onion powder

2 tbsp fresh parsley, chopped

½ tsp salt

¼ tsp pepper

Chicken:

4 (6-oz / 170-g) chicken breasts

Salt and freshly ground pepper, to taste

1 oz (28 g) butter, for frying

Herb butter:

4 oz (113 g) butter, at room temperature

1 garlic clove

½ tsp garlic powder

1 tbsp fresh parsley, finely chopped

1 tsp lemon juice

½ tsp salt

Directions:

Preheat the oven to 350°F (180°C). Cut the zucchini lengthwise into equal slices, half an inch thick. Pat dry with paper towels or a clean kitchen towel, and place on a baking tray lined with parchment paper. Sprinkle salt on the zucchini and let stand for 10 minutes.

Bake for 20 minutes in the oven, or until the zucchini is tender. Transfer to a cooling rack from the oven. Dry more if needed.

Put the butter in the saucepan over medium heat. Cut the mushrooms; put them in and stir fry well. Let cool.

Add the remaining ingredients for the zucchini roll-ups to a bowl except a third of the shredded cheese. Add the mushrooms and blend well.

Place a large amount of cheese on top of each zucchini slice.

Roll up and put inside the baking dish with seams down; sprinkle on top the remainder of the cheese.

Raise the temperature to 400°F (205°C). Bake for 20 minutes, or until the cheese turns bubbly and golden.

In the meantime, season your chicken and fry it over medium heat in butter until it is crispy outside and well cooked.

Herb butter:

To prepare the herb butter, mix the butter, garlic, garlic powder, fresh parsley, lemon juice, and salt thoroughly in a small bowl. Let sit for 30 minutes and serve on top of the chicken and zucchini roll-ups.

Nutrition: Calories: 913; Fat: 84 g; Carbs: 10 g; Fiber: 3g; Protein: 30 g

8 Keto Buffalo Drumsticks With Chili Aioli And Garlic

Preparation time: 10 minutes

Cooking time: 40 minutes

Servings: 4

Ingredients:

2 lb (907 g) chicken drumsticks or chicken wings

⅓ cup mayonnaise, keto-friendly

1 tbsp smoked paprika powder or smoked chili powder

1 garlic clove, minced

2 tbsp olive oil, and more for greasing the baking dish

2 tbsp white wine vinegar

1 tsp salt

1 tsp paprika powder

1 tbsp Tabasco

Directions:

Preheat the oven to 450°F (235°C).

Make the chili aioli: Combine the mayonnaise, smoked paprika powder, garlic clove, olive oil white wine vinegar, salt, paprika powder, and Tabasco for the marinade in a small bowl.

Put the drumsticks in a plastic bag, and pour the chili aioli into the plastic bag. Shake the bag thoroughly and let marinate for 10 minutes at room temperature.

Coat a baking dish with olive oil. Place the drumsticks in the baking dish and let bake in the preheated oven for 30 to 40 minutes or until they are done and have turned a nice color.

Remove the chicken wings from the oven and serve warm.

Nutrition: Calories: 570; Fat: 39 g; Carbs: 3 g; Fiber: 1 g; Protein: 43 g

9   Mustard-Thyme Chicken with Mushrooms

Preparation Time: 10 minutes

Cooking Time: 30 minutes

Servings: 4

Ingredients:

4 chicken thighs and 4 drumsticks

2 tbsp butter

2 tbsp olive oil

1 lb (450g) sliced brown or button mushrooms

½ finely chopped onion

1 minced garlic clove

1 cup white wine

½ cup chicken stock

1 tbsp chopped fresh thyme

1 tbsp Dijon mustard

½ cup heavy cream

½ cup grated parmesan cheese

Salt and pepper to taste

Directions:

Take a large pan and melt the butter and olive oil over medium-high heat.

Place the chicken in the pan and brown on both sides, about 4 minutes on each side. Remove the chicken from the pan and set aside.

Add sliced mushrooms, onion, and garlic to the pan. Sauté for a few minutes until mushrooms are slightly limp.

Add the white wine, chicken stock, and thyme, scraping up all the bits in the bottom of the pan.

Add chicken back to pan and simmer, uncovered, for about 15-20 minutes.

Stir in the Dijon mustard, cream, and parmesan cheese. When the cheese has melted, and the sauce has come together, season to taste with salt and pepper.

Quick Tip: Dijon mustard makes so many dishes so delicious; even King Louis XI didn't travel without mustard. Peppercorns are the most used spice in the United States, and mustard comes in second. So here's a quick tip: Dijon mustard works as an emulsifier in vinaigrette, meaning it helps the oil blend into vinegar without separating.

Nutrition: Fat: 39 g; Protein: 36 g; Carbs: 8 g; Fiber: 2 g; Calories: 520

10   Chicken Francese

Preparation Time: 10 minutes

Cooking Time: 25 minutes

Servings: 2

Ingredients:

2 medium-sized boneless and skinless chicken breasts, cut in half horizontally to make 4 fillets

2 eggs

1/4 cup finely grated parmesan cheese

2 tbsp fresh lemon juice

¼ cup almond flour

2 tbsp butter

4 tbsp olive oil

4 crushed garlic cloves

½ cup dry white wine

1 cup chicken stock

¼ cup fresh parsley chopped

1 cup heavy cream

Salt and pepper to taste

Directions:

Start with the sauce. While it is reducing, you can start with the chicken.

For the sauce:

Take a medium-sized pan on medium heat and add 1 tablespoon olive oil. Add the crushed garlic, and cook until fragrant. Add in the white wine, chicken stock, and parsley. Let it reduce to about a third, stirring occasionally. Reduce the heat and add the cream. Simmer on low heat until slightly thickened.

Add salt and pepper to taste to the sauce.

For the chicken:

If the chicken breasts are not even in thickness, flatten them with a meat hammer.

In a medium-sized bowl, whisk together eggs, parmesan cheese, lemon juice, salt, and black pepper.

Place the almond flour in a shallow bowl.

Add butter and 3 tablespoons olive oil into a medium-sized pan and put it over medium to hot heat. Place one chicken fillet in the almond flour flip over to coat both sides. Then place the chicken in the egg mixture and coat it thoroughly. Place the chicken in the heated pan and fry for about 4 minutes on each side until golden brown, or until it is cooked through.

Pace the chicken on a plate and drizzle over the sauce. Garnish with a dash of parsley.

Quick Tip: If you do not like almond flour, you can substitute it with coconut flour.

Nutrition: Fat: 99 g; Protein: 75 g; Carbs: 12 g; Fiber: 1.5 g; Calories: 1292

Side Dishes & Snacks

1 Baked Carrot with Bacon

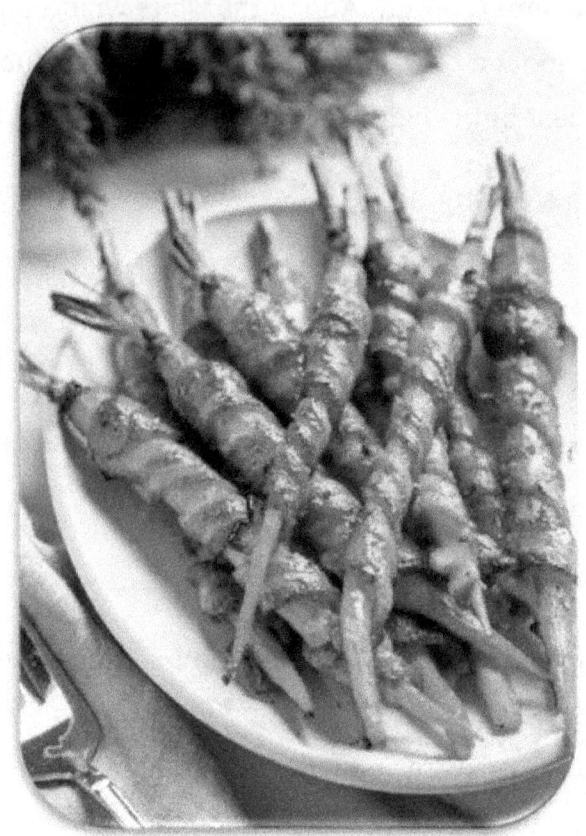

Preparation Time: 10 minutes

Cooking Time: 35 minutes

Servings: 4

Ingredients:

1½ lb carrots, peeled

12 slices bacon

1 tbsp black pepper

⅓ cup maple syrup

1 pinch parsley

Directions:

Preheat the oven to 400°F.

Wrap the bacon slices around your carrots from top to bottom. Add black pepper, sprinkle with maple syrup, and bake for about 20-25 minutes.

Top with parsley and serve.

Nutrition: Carbohydrates: 16 g; Fat: 26 g; Protein:10 g; Calories: 421

2 Standard Greek Salad

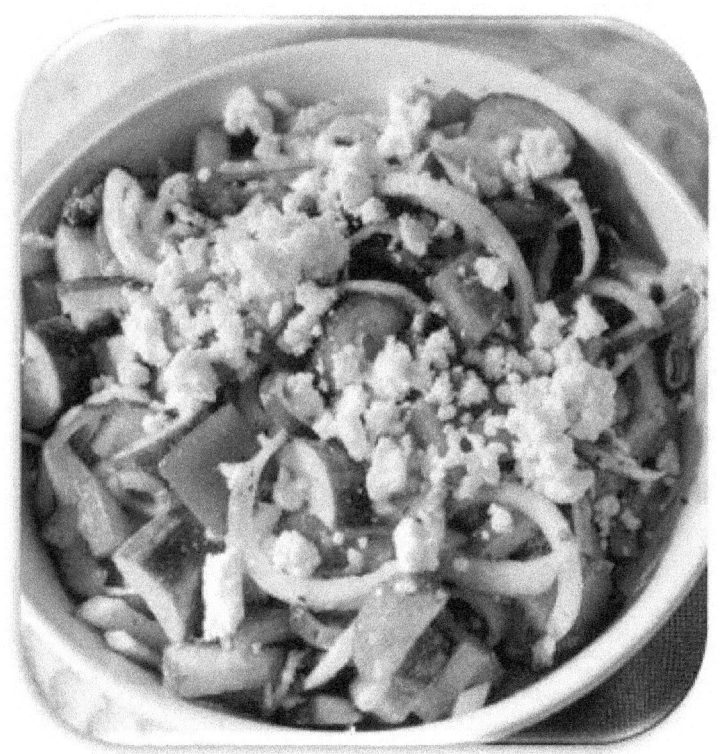

Preparation Time: 15 minutes

Cooking Time: 0 minutes

Servings: 4

Ingredients:

1 large tomato, cut into cubes

1 cucumber, sliced into half-moons

⅓ cup kalamata olives, halved

½ white onion, sliced

¾ cup feta, crumbled

2 tbsp red wine vinegar

2 tbsp lemon juice

1 tsp oregano, dried

Salt and pepper to taste

¼ cup extra-virgin olive oil

Directions:

In a separate bowl, combine the tomatoes, cucumbers, olives, and onion. Stir and top the mix with feta.

In another bowl, stir together the lemon juice, vinegar, oregano, salt, pepper, and olive oil. Gently whisk.

Sprinkle the salad with the dressing.

Nutrition: Carbohydrates: 7 g; Fat; 20 g; Protein; 5 g; Calories: 230

3 Creamy Mushrooms with Garlic and Thyme

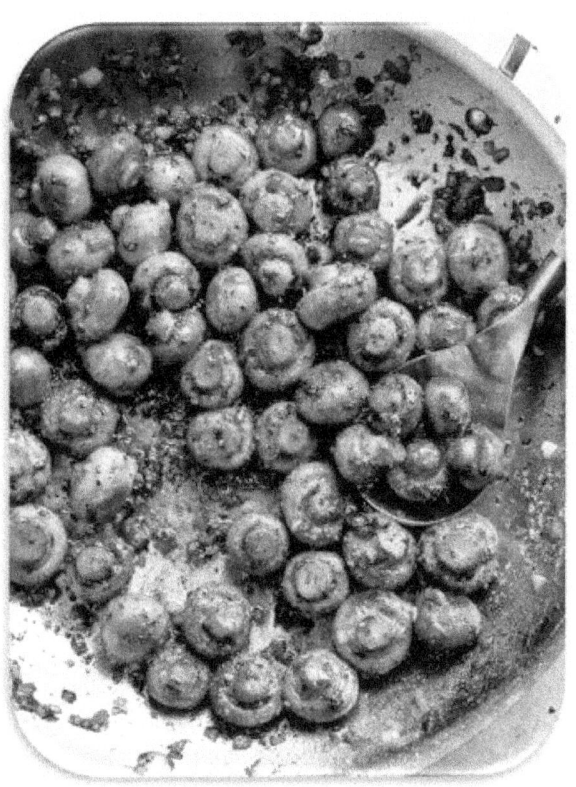

Preparation Time: 5 minutes

Cooking Time: 15 minutes

Servings: 4

Ingredients:

4 tbsp unsalted butter

½ cup onion, chopped

1 lb button mushrooms

2 tsp garlic, diced

1 tbsp fresh thyme

1 tbsp parsley, chopped

½ tsp salt

¼ tsp black pepper

Directions:

Melt the butter in a pan. Place the mushrooms into the pan. Add salt and pepper. Cook the mushroom mix for about 5 minutes until they're browned on both sides.

Add the garlic and thyme. Additionally, sauté the mushrooms for 1-2 minutes. Top them with parsley.

Nutrition: Carbohydrates: 45 g; Fat: 8 g; Protein: 3 g; Calories: 99

4 Easy Roasted Broccoli

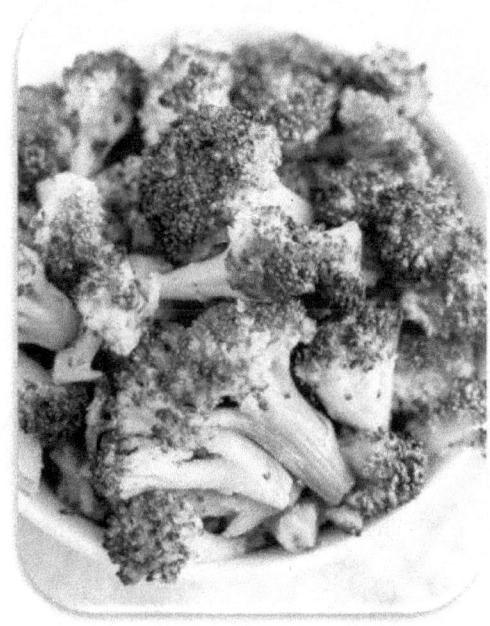

Preparation Time: 2 minutes

Cooking Time: 19 minutes

Servings: 4

Ingredients:

1 lb frozen broccoli, cut into florets

3 tsp olive oil

Sea salt to taste

Directions:

Place broccoli florets on a baking sheet greased with oil and put it in the oven (preheated to 400°F). Sprinkle the olive oil over the florets.

Cook for 12 minutes. Whisk well and bake for an additional 7 minutes.

Nutrition: Carbohydrates: 8 g; Fat: 3 g; Protein: 3 g; Calories: 58

5 Roasted Cabbage with Bacon

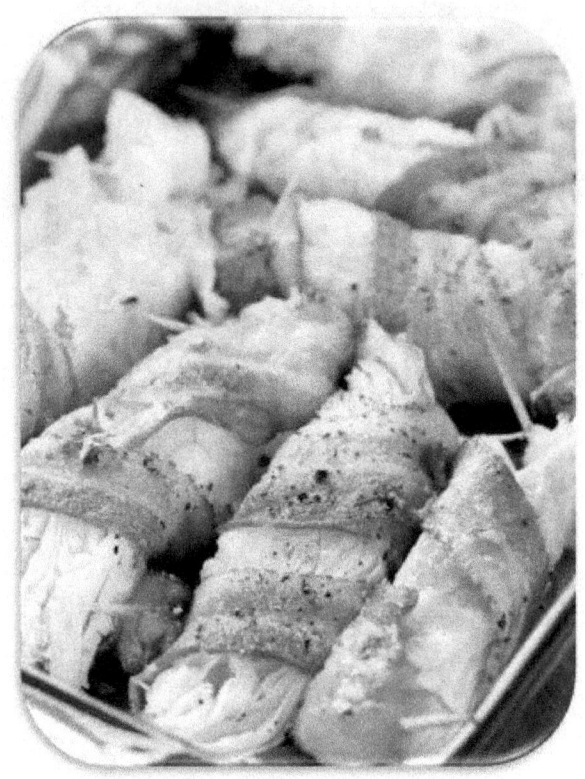

Preparation Time: 10 minutes

Cooking Time: 40 minutes

Servings: 4

Ingredients:

½ head cabbage, quartered

8 slices bacon, cut into thick pieces

¼ cup parmesan cheese, grated

1 tsp garlic powder

Salt and pepper to taste

1 pinch parsley, chopped

Directions:

Lightly sprinkle the cabbage wedges with the garlic powder and parmesan cheese. Wrap 2 pieces of bacon around each cabbage wedge.

Place your wrapped cabbage wedges on the baking sheet and put into the oven preheated to 350°F oven. Bake for 35-40 minutes. Top with parsley.

Nutrition: Carbohydrates: 7 g; Fat: 19 g: Protein: 9 g; Calories – 236

6 Baked Radish Snack

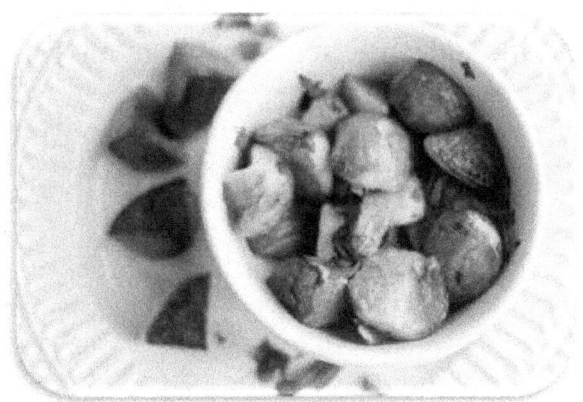

Preparation Time: 8 minutes

Cooking Time: 22 minutes

Servings: 2

Ingredients:

8 oz red radishes, washed and trimmed

2 tbsp olive oil

2 tbsp unsalted butter

1 clove garlic, diced

1 tsp lemon juice

¼ tsp oregano, dried

Salt and pepper to taste

1 pinch parsley

Directions:

Place the halved or quartered radishes into a separate bowl. Drizzle over the olive oil and add oregano. Stir gently.

Put the radish on the baking sheet and place it in the oven (preheated to 450°F).

Bake for 18-22 minutes. Mix a few times while baking.

Melt the butter in a saucepan. Add garlic and cook for about 3-5 minutes.

Remove your roasted radishes from the oven, sprinkle them with lemon juice, and top with the butter mix.

Nutrition: Carbohydrates: 4 g; Fat: 17 g; Protein:1 g; Calories: 164

7 Boiled Asparagus with Sliced Lemon

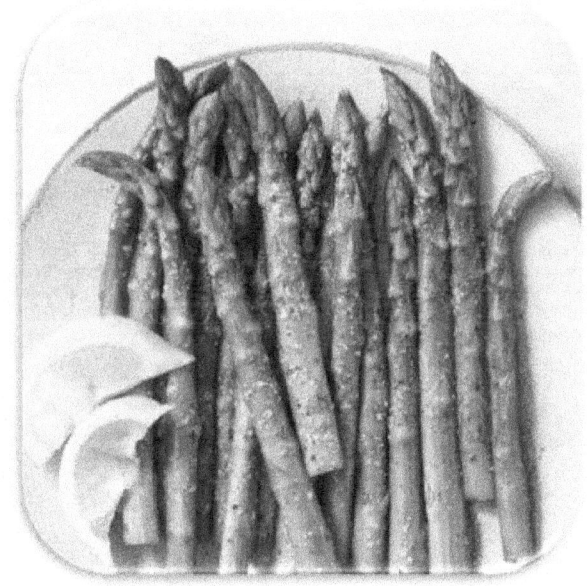

Preparation Time: 5 minutes

Cooking Time: 7 minutes

Servings: 1

Ingredients:

10 large asparagus

3 tbsp avocado oil

¼ tbsp lemon juice

2-3 pieces lemon

¼ cup water

½ tsp salt

Directions:

Place the asparagus in a pot of water. Boil for about 5-7 minutes.

Take the asparagus out of the pot. Sprinkle with lemon juice, avocado oil, and salt. Serve with the pieces of lemon.

Nutrition: Carbohydrates: 10.7 g; Fat: 43 g; Protein: 4.7 g; Calories: 447

8 Stuffed Eggs with Bacon-Avocado Filling

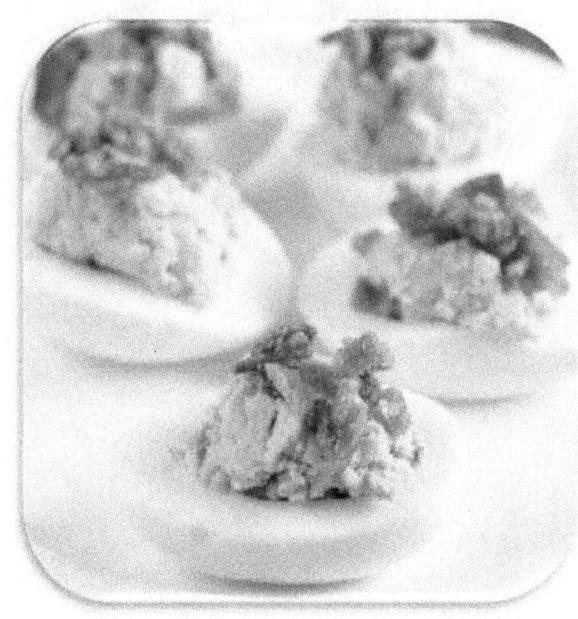

Preparation Time: 10 minutes

Cooking Time: 10 minutes

Servings: 1

Ingredients:

2 eggs, boiled and halved

1 tbsp mayonnaise

¼ tsp mustard

⅛ lemon, squeezed

¼ tsp garlic powder

⅛ tsp salt

⅛ tsp smoked paprika

¼ avocado

16 small pieces of bacon

Directions:

Fry the bacon for 3 minutes in a pan. Add the avocado and fry for an another 3 minutes (on lower heat).

Combine the mayonnaise, mustard, lemon, garlic powder, and salt in a separate bowl. Stir well.

Remove the yolk from the halved eggs and fill the egg halves with the mayonnaise mix. Top with the bacon-avocado filling.

Nutrition: Carbohydrates: 4 g; Fat: 30 g; Protein: 16 g; Calories: 342

9 Crab Cakes with Almond Flour

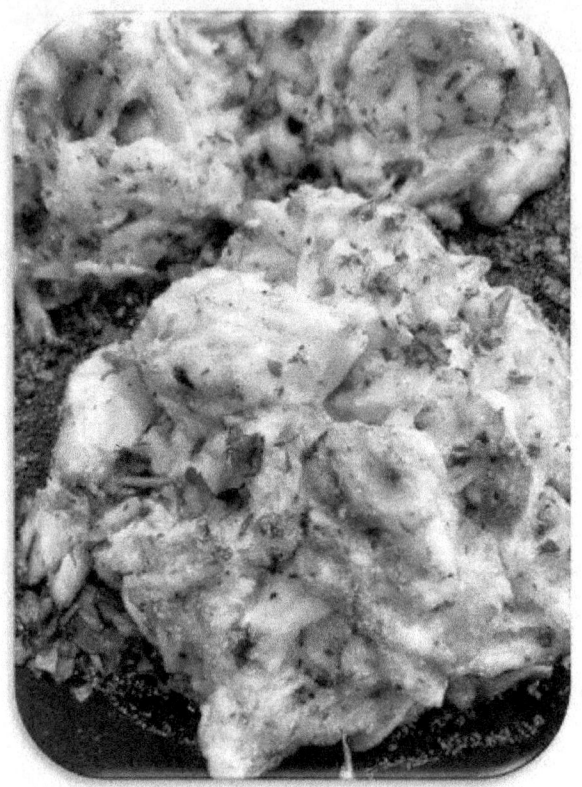

Preparation Time: 1 hour 10 minutes

Cooking Time: 15 minutes

Servings: 4

Ingredients:

8 oz fresh crab meat, shells removed

1 tbsp garlic, minced

¼ cup parsley, chopped

1 egg, slightly beaten

1 tbsp avocado oil

Mayonnaise

1 tbsp mustard

½ tsp kosher salt

½ tsp dried thyme

⅛ tsp cayenne pepper

½ cup almond flour

2 tbsp butter, for frying

Directions:

In a separate bowl, combine the crabmeat, garlic, parsley, egg, mayonnaise, mustard, kosher salt, thyme, cayenne pepper, and almond flour. Stir well. Form 4 cakes and place them into a fridge for 1 hour.

Melt the butter in the pan and put in your crab cakes. Fry for about 5-7 minutes on each side.

Nutrition: Carbohydrates: 4 g; Fat:17 g; Protein:13 g; Calories: 219

Spicy Zucchini Chips

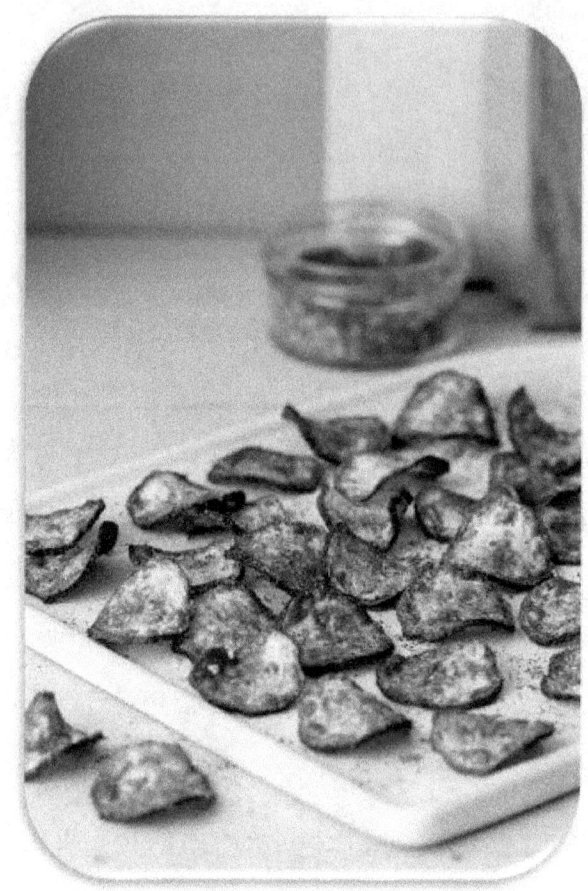

Preparation Time: 5 minutes

Cooking Time: 5 minutes

Servings: 4

Ingredients:

1 large zucchini, finely sliced

1 tbsp taco seasoning

Coconut oil, for frying

Salt to taste

Directions:

Wet the zucchini slices and sprinkle them with salt. Leave for 5 minutes.

Put the sliced zucchini into the frying pan and fry for 1-3 minutes on each side.

Top the fried slices with taco seasoning and enjoy your snack.

Nutrition: Carbohydrates: 23.3 g; Fat: 6 12 g; Protein: 0.2 g; Calories: 164

11 Cucumber Salad with Tomatoes and Feta

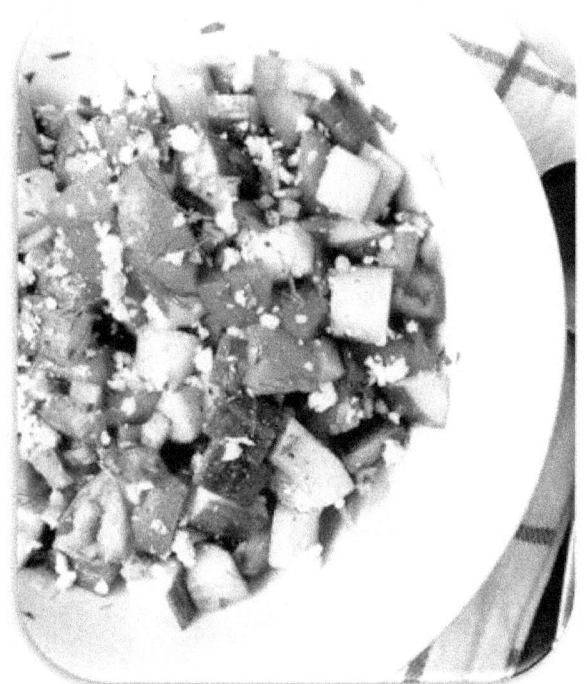

Preparation Time: 15 minutes

Cooking Time: 0 minutes

Servings: 4

Ingredients:

2 cucumbers, diced

6 tomatoes, diced

¾ cup feta cheese, crumbled

½ white onion, chopped

1 garlic clove, minced

2 tbsp lime juice

2 tbsp parsley, chopped

2 tbsp dill, chopped

3 tbsp olive oil

3 tbsp red wine vinegar

Salt and black pepper, to taste

Directions:

Combine all the ingredients in a bowl.

Stir thoroughly and serve.

Nutrition: Carbohydrates: 5 g; Fat: 10 g; Protein: 3 g; Calories: 125

Salads Recipes

1 Artichoke and Avocado Pasta Salad

Preparation Time: 10 minutes

Cooking Time: 30 minutes

Servings: 10

Ingredients:

2 cups spiral pasta (uncooked)

¼ cup Romano cheese (grated)

1 can (14 oz.) of artichoke hearts (coarsely chopped and drained well)

1 avocado (medium-sized, ripe, cubed)

2 plum tomatoes (chopped coarsely)

For the dressing:

1 tbsp fresh cilantro (chopped)

2 tbsp lime juice

¼ cup canola oil

1½ tsp lime zest (grated)

½ tsp of pepper (freshly ground)

½ tsp of kosher salt

Directions:

Follow the directions mentioned on the package for cooking the pasta. Drain it and rinse using cold water.

Then, take a large-sized bowl and in it, add the pasta along with the tomatoes, artichoke hearts, cheese, and avocado. Combine them well. Then, take another bowl and add all the ingredients of the dressing to it. Whisk them together and, once combined, add the dressing over the pasta.

Gently toss the mixture to coat everything evenly in the dressing and then refrigerate.

Nutrition: Calories: 188; Protein: 6 g; Fat: 10 g; Carbs: 21 g; Fiber: 2 g

2 Apple Arugula and Turkey Salad in a Jar

Preparation Time: 20 minutes

Cooking Time: 0 minutes

Servings: 4

Ingredients:

3 tbsp red wine vinegar

2 tbsp chives (freshly minced)

½ cup orange juice

1-3 tbsp of sesame oil

¼ tsp pepper (coarsely ground)

¼ tsp of salt

For the salad:

4 tsp curry powder

4 cups of turkey (cubed, cooked)

4 cups of baby spinach or fresh arugula

1/4 tsp salt

½ tsp pepper (coarsely ground)

1 cup halved green grapes

1 apple (large-sized, chopped)

11 oz. mandarin oranges (properly drained)

1 tbsp lemon juice

½ cup walnuts (chopped)

½ cup dried cranberries or pomegranate seeds

Directions:

Take a small-sized bowl and, in it, add the first six ingredients from the list into it. Whisk them. Then take a large bowl and in it, add the turkey and the seasonings. Toss the turkey cubes to coat them with the seasoning. Take another bowl and in it, add the lemon juice and toss the apple chunks in the juice.

Take four jars and divide the layers in the order I mention here - first goes the orange juice mixture, the second layer is the turkey, then apple, oranges, grapes, cranberries or pomegranate seeds, walnuts, and spinach or arugula. Cover the jars and then refrigerate them.

Nutrition: Calories: 471; Protein: 45 g; Fat: 19 g; Carbs: 33 g; Fiber: 5g

3 Summertime Slaw

Preparation Time: 35 minutes

Cooking Time: 15 minutes

Servings: 10-12

Ingredients:

1/3 cup canola oil

¾ cup white vinegar

¾ cup sugar

1 tsp pepper

1 tsp salt

1 tbsp water

½ tsp red pepper flakes (crushed and optional)

2 tomatoes (medium-sized, seeded, peeled, and chopped)

1 pack of coleslaw mix (fourteen oz.)

1 sweet red pepper (small-sized, chopped)

1 green pepper (small-sized, chopped)

1 onion (large-sized, chopped)

½ cup of sweet pickle relish

Directions:

Take a saucepan of large size and in it, combine water, sugar, oil, vinegar, pepper, salt, and if you want, then red pepper flakes too. Cook them over medium heat by continuously stirring the mixture. Keep stirring until it comes to a boil. Cook for another two minutes or so, and make sure that all the sugar has dissolved. Once done, cool the mixture to room temperature by stirring it.

In a large salad bowl, combine the pickle relish, coleslaw mix, peppers, onion, and tomatoes. On top of the mixture, add the dressing and toss the mixture to coat it properly. Cover the mixture and put it in the refrigerator for a night.

Nutrition: Calories: 138; Protein: 1 g; Fat: 6 g; Carbs: 21g; Fiber: 2g

4 Zucchini and Tomato Spaghetti

Preparation Time: 25 minutes

Cooking Time: 5 minutes

Servings: 4

Ingredients:

2 large-sized zucchini, nicely spiralized

3 cups red and yellow cherry tomatoes

4 oz. spaghetti (whole wheat – optional)

Toppings – grated parmesan

For the avocado sauce:

¼ cup of olive oil

1 avocado

½ cup of parsley (fresh)

½ tsp salt

3-4 green onions (only the green parts)

1 lemon (juiced)

1 clove of garlic

A pinch of pepper (freshly ground)

Directions:

Firstly, take all the ingredients of the sauce and pulse them so that they are combined well and form a smooth mixture. Set it aside.

Then, follow the directions mentioned in the package for cooking the spaghetti. Drain the cooked spaghetti and keep it aside too.

Take a large-sized skillet and heat the cherry tomatoes in it. Use a bit of olive oil. Keep cooking the tomatoes until they seem well-roasted. They will seem loosened with their skins split. Once done, remove the tomatoes from the flame and set aside.

Then, add the zucchini to the same skillet. Stir and toss for about two minutes until they look crisp. Then, add the avocado sauce and the spaghetti. Keep tossing until everything has been properly combined. Season with pepper and salt as per taste. Top with parmesan and the tomatoes that you had reserved earlier.

Note: If you want to make this super-healthy, you can stick only to the zucchini and skip the pasta altogether. When the tomatoes are cooking, keep the lid covered because the hot oil tends to splatter.

Nutrition: Calories: 330 | Protein: 7.1 g | Fat: 20 g | Carbs: 35.3 g | Fiber: 8 g

5 White Bean Salad

Preparation Time: 5 minutes

Cooking Time: 5 minutes

Servings: 4

Ingredients:

For the salad:

2 green peppers, coarsely chopped

½ cup chopped cucumber

½ cup chopped tomatoes

1½ cups white beans (boiled)

¼ cup green onions (chopped)

¼ cup fresh dill (chopped)

¼ cup parsley (chopped)

4 eggs (hard-boiled)

For the dressing:

1 tbsp lemon juice

1 tsp vinegar

2 tbsp olive oil

1 tsp Sumac

1/2 tsp salt

For quick onion pickle:

1 tsp sumac

1 tsp salt

1 tsp vinegar

1 tbsp lemon juice

2 thinly sliced red onions (medium-sized)

2 cups water (hot)

Directions:

Take a large-sized bowl and add all the salad ingredients in it, keeping the eggs aside.

In case you do not want to pickle the onions, you can simply make thin slices and then mix them with the other ingredients. But, if you do want to pickle the onions, then continue with it before you move on to the dressing. The recipe for the onions is mentioned later.

Take all the ingredients of the dressing together in one bowl and whisk them together. Then, drizzle the dressing over the salad. Toss well, and on the top, place the halved eggs.

For the pickled onions:

First, take very hot water and place the sliced onions in it. Blanch the onions for one minute and then immediately transfer them into a pot of very cold water so that the cooking stops. Let them stay in that pot of cold water for a few minutes. Once done, drain them well.

Mix sumac, lemon juice, salt, and vinegar, and then pour the mixture over the onion that you just drained. Keep it for five to ten minutes.

Then, add the onions into the mixture of salad and stir well. Keep some onions aside so that you can use them as a topping.

Nutrition: Calories: 449; Protein: 23.6 g; Fat: 23.3 g; Carbs: 39.7 g

6 Lentil Bolognese

Preparation Time: 20 minutes

Cooking Time: 40 minutes

Servings: 4-6

Ingredients:

2 boxes penne pasta

1 onion (medium-sized, finely chopped)

1 red bell pepper (finely chopped)

2 tbsp olive oil

2 carrots (large-sized, sliced)

4 cloves of garlic (large ones, minced)

1 tbsp of miso

1 tsp pepper

1 tsp salt

4 cups water

1 can tomato paste (measuring 5½ oz)

1 cup brown lentils (dried)

1 cup cherry tomatoes (halved)

Toppings (optional) – black pepper, sage leaves, parmesan (grated)

Directions:

Take a large-sized skillet and start by heating the oil in it on a medium flame. Then, add the chopped onions. In about five minutes, they will soften and appear to be translucent. Then, add the red pepper, carrots, sugar, and sea salt to the skillet and keep cooking. Stir the mixture from time to time. In fifteen minutes, everything will be well caramelized. Then, add the tomato paste and the garlic and let the mixture cook for three minutes or until you get a caramelized fragrance from the paste.

Then, add the lentils, miso, and water to the skillet and bring the mixture to a boil. Once the mixture is boiling, reduce the flame and keep the skillet uncovered while the lentils are cooking. This will take about 25-30 minutes. Keep stirring the lentils from time to time, and in case they look dry, add some water. After that, add the cherry tomatoes and keep stirring.

While you are cooking the lentils, take a large pot and fill it with water. Add a generous amount of salt and bring the water to a boil. Then, add the chickpea pasta into the water and cook it for about five to six minutes or until al dente. Don't overcook it. Once done, drain the water and set aside to cool.

Divide the penne into 4-6 meal prep containers and top with bolognese. Sprinkle a few sage leaves or a bit of parmesan if you want.

Nutrition: Calories: 486 | Protein: 29.3 g | Fat: 9 g | Carbs: 78.2 g | Fiber: 15 g

7 Kale, Lemon, and White Bean Soup

Preparation Time: 25 minutes

Cooking Time: 1 hour 30 minutes

Servings: 2

Ingredients:

150 grams dried cannellini beans

2 cups vegetable stock

5 cups water

1 white onion (large-sized, diced)

2 tbsp olive oil

8 cloves of garlic

Kombu (one-inch strip)

1 tsp dried thyme

2 potatoes (small ones, cubed after peeling)

2 bay leaves

1 cup kale

1 lemon (juiced and zest)

Directions:

Take an ample amount of water to soak the dried beans and keep them soaked for about twelve hours. Drain the beans properly; they should become double their size. Rinse them. They are ready to be cooked.

Take a large-sized pot, and in it, add one tablespoon of oil and heat it. Then, add the diced onion to the pot and cook the onions until they become golden and soft.

Then, add the stock and water along with garlic, dried beans, kombu, thyme, and bay leaves. Keep the pot covered and then bring it to a boil. Once it starts boiling, reduce the flame to a simmer and wait for about forty minutes.

While it is cooking, start with the kale. Wash it thoroughly. All the tough inner stalks should be removed. Then, start slicing them into ribbons of one-inch thickness. It looks good when you have delicate small pieces, so you should take your time with this.

After about half an hour, add the potatoes to the pot and then let the preparation simmer for ten more minutes. After this, both the potatoes and the beans should be soft. Take out the kombu and bay leaves. Take a potato masher and use it carefully to mash at least half of the beans and potatoes.

Add the kale. Cook the mixture for ten more minutes. The water content needs to be checked now and see whether it is right or whether it needs to be topped up a bit. If the water is too much, then cook uncovered for a few minutes so that it dries up.

Once you notice the kale softening, add a tablespoon of olive oil to the pot. Stir in the zest and lemon juice as well, and your dish is ready.

Nutrition: Calories: 574 | Protein: 22 g | Fat: 16 g | Carbs: 106 g | Fiber: 23 g

8 Broccoli Quinoa Casserole

Preparation Time: 20 minutes

Cooking Time: 45 minutes

Servings: 5

Ingredients:

4 ½ cups vegetable stock

2 ½ cups quinoa (uncooked)

½ tsp salt

2 tbsp pesto

2 tsp cornstarch

12 oz mozzarella cheese (skimmed)

2 cups spinach (fresh and organic)

1/3 cup parmesan cheese

3 medium-sized green onions (chopped)

12 oz broccoli florets (fresh)

Directions:

Set the temperature of the oven to 400°F and preheat. Take a rectangular baking dish and add the quinoa to it along with the green onions. In the meantime, take a large-sized bowl and add the broccoli florets to it. Microwave the florets at high for about five minutes. Once done, set them aside.

Take a large-sized mixing bowl and in it, add the pesto, vegetable sauce, cornstarch, and salt. Use a wire whisk to mix all of them properly. Now, heat this mixture until it starts to boil. You can either do this in the microwave, or you can use your stovetop as well.

Now, take the vegetable stock and the spinach and add them to the quinoa. Add three-quarter of the mozzarella cheese and the parmesan as well. Bake the mixture for 30-35 minutes. Once done, take the casserole of quinoa out and then mix the broccoli into it. Take the rest of the cheese and sprinkle on top. Place the preparation back in the oven for another five minutes. By this time, all the cheese will melt.

Nutrition: Calories: 491 | Protein: 27.6 g | Fat: 16 g | Carbs: 61.3 g | Fiber: 9 g

9 Creamy Chicken Salad

Preparation Time: 10 minutes

Cooking Time: 30 minutes

Servings: 4

Ingredients:

1 lb chicken breast

2 avocados

2 garlic cloves

3 tbsp lime juice

1/3 cup onion

1 minced jalapeno pepper

A dash of salt

1 tbsp cilantro

A dash of pepper

Directions:

If you like traditional chicken salad, this is an excellent alternative to help provide healthier fats along with a good chunk of protein. You will want to start this recipe off by prepping the oven to 400°F.

As this warms up, get out your cooking sheet and line it with paper or foil. Next, it is time to get out the chicken. Layer the chicken breast with some olive oil before seasoning to your liking. I generally use salt and pepper, but feel free to use anything like garlic or onion powder! When the chicken is all set, you will want to line the pieces along the surface of your cooking sheet. Pop it into the oven for about 20 minutes. By the end, the chicken should be cooked through and can be taken out of the oven for chilling. Once cool enough to handle, either dice or shred your chicken depending on how you like your chicken salad.

Now that your chicken is all cooked, it is time to assemble your salad! You can begin this process by adding everything into a bowl and mashing down the avocado. Sprinkle some salt over the top and serve immediately. Whether you like your chicken salad straight out of the bowl or in a low-carb wrap, it can be enjoyed in several different ways!

Nutrition: Fats: 20 g; Carbs: 4 g; Proteins: 25 g

10   Simple Tuna Salad

Preparation Time: 5 minutes

Cooking Time: 0 minutes

Servings: 4

Ingredients:

10 oz canned tuna, drained

1 avocado, chopped

1 rib celery, chopped

2 cloves fresh garlic, minced

3 tbsp mayonnaise

1 red onion chopped

1 tbsp lemon juice

8 sprigs parsley

¼ cucumber, chopped

Salt and pepper to taste

Directions:

Divide the parsley into two halves. Mix all the ingredients except half of the parsley in a separate bowl. Stir well. Add salt and pepper to taste. Top with the remaining parsley.

Nutrition: Carbohydrates: 1.7 g; Fat:16.3 g; Protein: 13.9 g; Calories: 225

Soup Recipes

1 Egg Drop Soup

Dairy-Free, Nut-Free, One-Pot, Under 30 Minutes

This egg drop soup captures the flavor of your favorite Chinese takeout without all the carbs that would normally make it off-limits. The broth presents with full flavors of ginger and white pepper but is still incredibly simple to make.

Preparation Time: 2 minutes

Cooking Time: 10 minutes

Servings: 2

Ingredients:

4 cups chicken broth

1 tsp pink Himalayan sea salt

½ tsp ground ginger

½ tsp toasted sesame oil

Pinch of ground white pepper

2 large eggs

1 scallion, both white and green parts, sliced

Directions:

In a medium saucepan, combine the broth, salt, ginger, sesame oil, and white pepper. Cook over medium-high heat until the soup is boiling.

In a small bowl, lightly beat the eggs.

Stirring the soup in a circular motion, slowly drizzle the beaten egg into the center of the vortex. When all the egg is mixed in, stop stirring.

Cook for an additional 2 minutes, until the egg is cooked through. Then pour into 2 bowls. Sprinkle with the scallions and serve.

Cooking Tip: This soup is thinner than other egg drop soups you may have had. This is because most restaurants thicken the soup with cornstarch. If you want a similar texture, mix ½ tsp xanthan gum with ½ cup water until smooth, then stir it into the soup to thicken it.

Nutrition: Calories: 121; Total Fat: 8 g; Protein: 10 g; Total Carbohydrates: 3 g; Fiber: 0 g; Erythritol: 0 g; Net Carbs: 3 g

2 Beef Chili

Egg-Free, Nut-Free, One-Pot

Whether it's for a cold winter night or a summer barbecue outdoors, chili is the perfect dish. This keto chili doesn't skimp on the flavor, either. It provides a nice balance of heat and acidity but can be easily modified to fit any taste buds. Serve it in bowls topped with cheese, or spread it on hot dogs to create the perfect keto chili dogs. No matter how you choose to eat it, you won't likely find yourself missing chili again.

Preparation Time: 5 minutes

Cooking Time: 50 minutes

Servings: 4

Instructions:

½ green bell pepper, cored, seeded, and chopped

½ medium onion, chopped

2 tbsp extra-virgin olive oil

1 tbsp minced garlic

1 lb ground beef (80/20)

1 (14-oz) can crushed tomatoes

1 cup beef broth

1 tbsp ground cumin

1 tbsp chili powder

2 tsp paprika

1 tsp pink Himalayan sea salt

¼ tsp cayenne pepper

Directions:

In a medium pot, combine the bell pepper, onion, and olive oil. Cook over medium heat for 8 to 10 minutes, until the onion is translucent.

Add the garlic and cook for 1 minute longer, until fragrant.

Add the ground beef and cook for 7 to 10 minutes, until browned.

Add the tomatoes, broth, cumin, chili powder, paprika, salt, and cayenne. Stir to combine.

Simmer the chili for 30 minutes, until the flavors come together, then enjoy.

Variation Tip: If you allow soy in your keto diet, black soybeans are actually very low in carbs and can be added to this recipe to make it a chili with beans.

Nutrition: Calories: 406; Total Fat: 31 g; Protein: 22 g; Total Carbohydrates: 12 g; Fiber: 4 g; Erythritol: 0 g; Net Carbs: 8 g

3 Broccoli Cheddar Soup

Egg-Free, Nut-Free, One-Pot, Under 30 Minutes

This classic soup could have easily been invented for the keto diet. It combines the nutrients of broccoli with the fat needed to keep you in ketosis. The result is a rich and cheesy soup with a fantastic broccoli flavor.

Preparation Time: 5 minutes

Cooking Time: 15 minutes

Servings: 2

Ingredients:

¼ medium onion, chopped

2 tbsp butter

1 garlic clove, minced

1 cup chicken broth

¾ tsp pink Himalayan salt

½ tsp freshly ground black pepper

¼ tsp dry mustard powder

8 oz fresh broccoli florets, cooked and finely chopped

1 cup heavy (whipping) cream

1 cup shredded cheddar cheese

Directions:

In a medium pot, combine the onion, butter, and garlic over medium heat. Cook for 7 to 10 minutes, until the onion is tender.

Add the broth, salt, pepper, and mustard, and bring the mixture to a boil.

Reduce the heat and add the broccoli and cream.

Slowly add the cheese, stirring.

The soup is ready to serve as soon as the cheese is melted and has blended with the rest of the soup.

Nutrition: Calories: 789; Total Fat: 75 g; Protein: 19 g; Total Carbohydrates: 14 g; Fiber: 4 g; Erythritol: 0 g; Net Carbs: 10 g

4 Loaded Cauliflower Soup

Egg-Free, Nut-Free, One-Pot

This is a ketogenic rendition of the classic baked potato soup. It's thick, creamy, and loaded with the flavors of your favorite baked potato toppings. The cauliflower is creamy, smooth, and practically indistinguishable from the potatoes that would traditionally be in this soup. For me, this dish is the ultimate comfort food.

Preparation Time: 5 minutes

Cooking Time: 25 minutes

Servings: 3

Ingredients:

2 bacon strips, roughly chopped

¼ medium onion, chopped

1½ cups chicken broth

1½ cups chopped cauliflower florets

½ tsp pink Himalayan salt

½ tsp freshly ground black pepper

¼ tsp garlic powder

1 cup heavy (whipping) cream

1 cup shredded cheddar cheese

3 tbsp sour cream

2 tbsp chopped fresh chives

Directions:

In a medium saucepan, cook the bacon over medium-high heat for 8 to 10 minutes, until crispy. Transfer the bacon to a paper towel-lined plate.

Add the onion to the saucepan and cook for 8 to 10 minutes, until tender.

Add the broth, cauliflower, salt, pepper, and garlic powder. Bring to a simmer and cook for about 5 minutes, until the cauliflower is tender.

Reduce the heat and stir in the cream. Slowly stir in the cheese.

Divide the soup among 3 serving bowls. Top each bowl with 1 tbsp of sour cream and equal portions of the bacon crumbles and chives.

Variation Tip: Kohlrabi is a great substitute for potatoes. To put a little different spin on this soup, try using kohlrabi instead of the cauliflower.

Nutrition: Calories: 510; Total Fat: 48 g; Protein: 15 g; Total Carbohydrates: 7 g; Fiber: 1 g; Erythritol: 0 g; Net Carbs: 6 g

5 Cabbage Soup with Beef

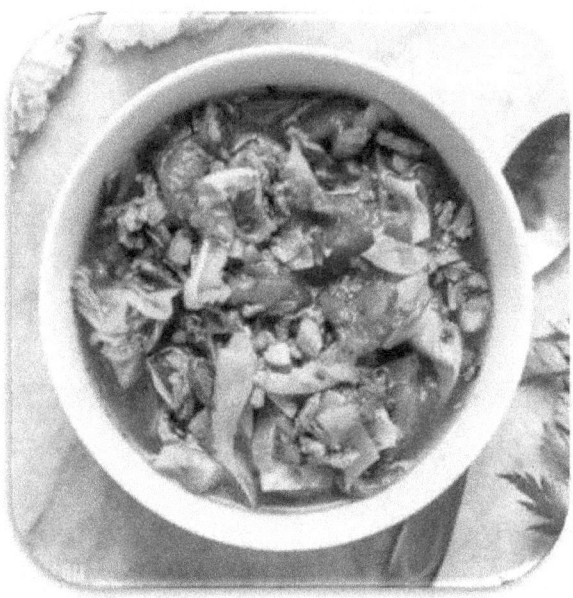

Preparation Time: 15 minutes

Cooking Time: 20 minutes

Servings: 4

Ingredients:

2 tbsp olive oil

1 medium onion, chopped

1 lb fillet steak, cut into pieces

½ stalk celery, chopped

1 carrot, peeled and diced

½ head small green cabbage, cut into pieces

2 cloves garlic, minced

4 cups beef broth

2 tbsp fresh parsley, chopped

1 tsp dried thyme

1 tsp dried rosemary

1 tsp garlic powder

Salt and black pepper to taste

Directions:

Heat oil in a pot (use medium heat). Add the beef and cook until it is browned. Put the onion into the pot and boil for 3-4 minutes.

Add the celery and carrot. Stir well and cook for about 3-4 minutes. Add the cabbage and boil until it starts softening. Add garlic and simmer for about 1 minute.

Pour the broth into the pot. Add the parsley and garlic powder. Mix thoroughly and reduce heat to medium-low.

Cook for 10-15 minutes.

Nutrition: Carbohydrates: 4 g; Fat: 11 g; Protein; 12 g; Calories –177

6 Cauliflower Rice Soup with Chicken

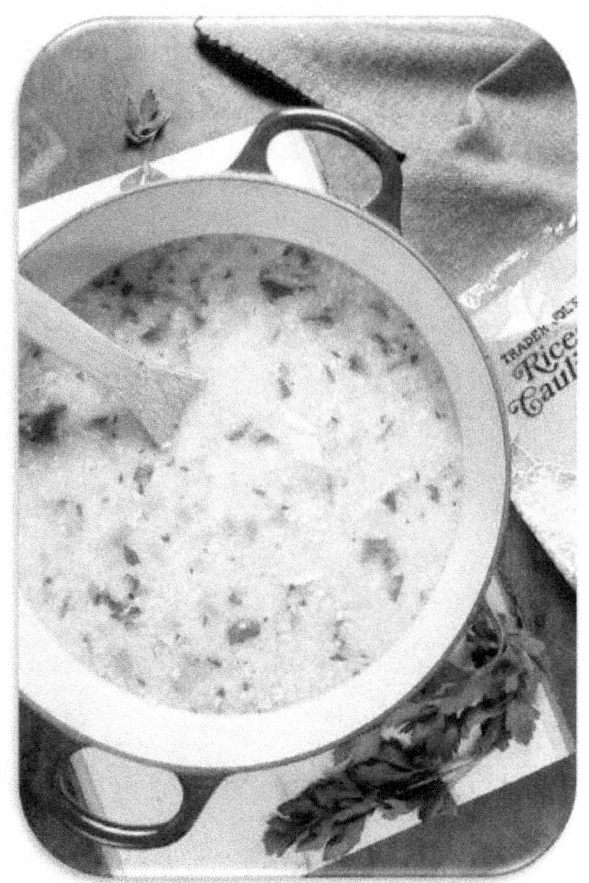

Preparation Time: 10 minutes

Cooking Time: 1 hour

Servings: 5

Ingredients:

2½ lbs chicken breasts, boneless and skinless

8 tbsp butter

¼ cup celery, chopped

½ cup onion, chopped

4 cloves garlic, minced

2 (12-oz) packages steamed cauliflower rice

1 tbsp parsley, chopped

2 tsp poultry seasoning

½ cup carrot, grated

¾ tsp rosemary

1 tsp salt

¾ tsp pepper

4 oz cream cheese

4¾ cup chicken broth

Directions:

Put shredded chicken breasts into a saucepan and pour in the chicken broth. Add salt and pepper. Cook for 1 hour.

In another pot, melt the butter. Add the onion, garlic, and celery. Sauté until the mix is translucent. Add the rice cauliflower, rosemary, and carrot. Mix and cook for 7 minutes.

Add the chicken breasts and broth to the cauliflower mix. Put the lid on and simmer for 15 minutes.

Nutrition: Carbohydrates: 6 g; Fat: 30 g; Protein: 27 g; Calories: 415

7 Quick Pumpkin Soup

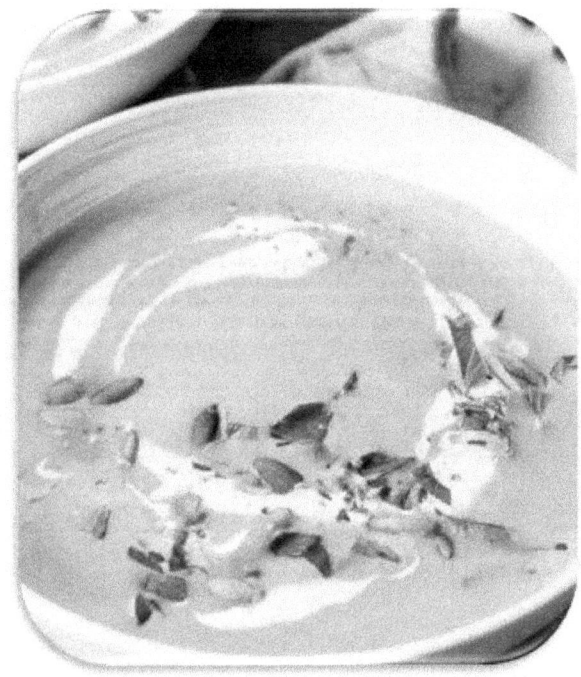

Preparation Time: 10 minutes

Cooking Time: 20 minutes

Servings: 4-6

Ingredients:

1 cup coconut milk

2 cups chicken broth

6 cups baked pumpkin

1 tsp garlic powder

1 tsp ground cinnamon

1 tsp dried ginger

1 tsp nutmeg

1 tsp paprika

Salt and pepper to taste

Sour cream or coconut yogurt, for topping

Pumpkin seeds, toasted, for topping

Directions:

Combine the coconut milk, broth, baked pumpkin, and spices in a soup pan (under medium heat). Stir occasionally and simmer for 15 minutes.

With an immersion blender, blend the soup mix for 1 minute.

Top with sour cream or coconut yogurt and pumpkin seeds.

Nutrition: Carbohydrates: 8.1 g; Fat: 9.8 g; Protein:3.1 g; Calories:123

8 Fresh Avocado Soup

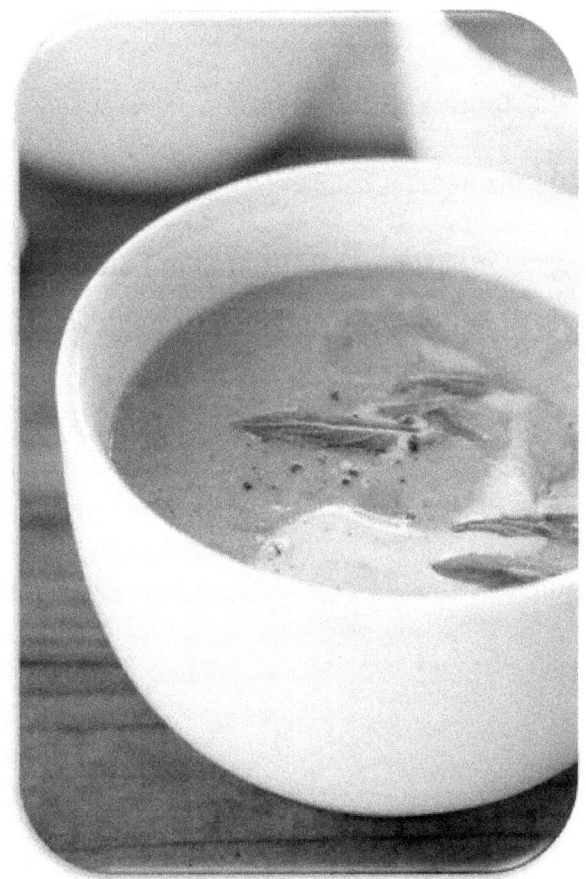

Preparation Time: 5 minutes

Cooking Time: 10 minutes

Servings: 2

Ingredients:

1 ripe avocado

2 romaine lettuce leaves, washed and chopped

1 cup coconut milk, chilled

1 tbsp lime juice

20 fresh mint leaves

Salt to taste

Directions:

Mix all your ingredients thoroughly in a blender.

Chill in the fridge for 5-10 minutes.

Nutrition: Carbohydrates: 12 g; Fat: 26 g; Protein: 4 g; Calories; 280

9 Simply Delicious Chicken Soup

Preparation Time: 5 minutes

Cooking Time: 50 minutes

Servings: 2

Ingredients:

3 chicken thighs

2 tbsp olive oil

2 tbsp butter

1/2 chopped onion

2 chopped celery stalks

2 crushed garlic cloves

1/2 tsp dried thyme

1/2 tsp paprika

4 cups chicken stock

Salt and pepper to taste

Directions:

Take a medium to large size pot. Add olive oil and butter, and bring to medium heat. Add the chicken and brown on all sides. Remove the chicken from the pot and set aside.

Add the onion, celery, and garlic to the pot and sauté for about 5 minutes.

Place the chicken back in the pot. Add the chicken stock as well as the thyme and paprika.

Place the lid on the pot (with a small opening, so it won't overcook) and let it cook for about 40 minutes. If there are bones in the chicken, remove them and cut the meat into bite-size pieces. Place the chicken back into the pot.

Season to taste with salt and pepper.

Quick Tip: For truly unforgettable chicken soup, simply add chicken feet. It doesn't sound too appealing; however, this adds a punch of flavor and will take your soup to the next level. Your nearest Asian grocery store should have them in stock.

Nutrition: Fat: 40 g; Protein: 26 g; Carbs: 8.5 g; Fiber: 1.4 g; Calories: 498

10   Reuben Soup

This unusual soup, based on the classic sandwich, might become your new favorite. It's salty, spicy, tart, and sweet, and the parsley adds an unexpected earthy flavor. Parsley is not just a topping, it also contains folate and several flavonoids such as luteolin, quercetin, and kaempferol that help protect cells from oxidative stress.

Preparation Time: 15 minutes

Cooking Time: 20 minutes

Servings: 4

1 Pan/Pot, 500 Calories Or Fewer, Nut-Free

Ingredients:

3 tbsp extra-virgin olive oil

1 onion, chopped

2 celery stalks, chopped

1 tbsp minced garlic

6 cups low-sodium beef broth

12 oz corned beef, chopped

2 cups sauerkraut

2 tbsp hot mustard

½ tsp caraway seeds

1½ cups shredded Swiss cheese

2 tbsp chopped fresh parsley, for garnish

Directions:

Heat the olive oil in a large stockpot over medium-high heat and sauté the onion, celery, and garlic until softened for about 5 minutes.

Stir in the beef broth, corned beef, sauerkraut, mustard, and caraway seeds and bring to a boil.

Reduce the heat to low and simmer until the vegetables are tender, about 15 minutes.

Serve topped with the Swiss cheese and parsley.

Cooking Tip: Reuben sandwiches are packed with layers of meat, tart sauerkraut, and melted Swiss cheese. Yum. The only element missing here is the bread, but caraway seeds evoke the taste of rye, so that should help.

Nutrition: Calories: 493; Total Fat: 38 g; Total Carbohydrates: 9 g; Net Carbs: 6 g; Fiber: 3 g; Protein: 30 g

Smoothies Recipes

1 Strawberry Avocado Smoothie

Preparation Time: 10 minutes

Cooking Time: 0 minutes

Servings: 4

Ingredients:

2 cups frozen strawberries

2 large avocados, peeled, pitted, chopped

3 cups almond milk, unsweetened

½ cup erythritol

Directions:

Take a high-powered blender and place the strawberries, avocado, almond milk, and erythritol into it.

Blend until smooth.

Pour into glasses and serve with crushed ice.

Nutrition: Calories: 106; Fat: 20 g; Carbohydrate: 6 g; Protein: 1 g

2 Chocolate Keto Smoothie

Preparation Time: 10 minutes

Cooking Time: 0 minutes

Servings: 1

Ingredients:

1 tsp plain whey protein or dark chocolate

¼ cup coconut milk or heavy whipping cream

2 tbsp coconut butter or almond butter or chia seeds

1 tbsp unsweetened cacao powder

½ cup ice + ¼ cup water

1 tbsp extra virgin coconut oil or MCT oil

3-5 drops Stevia extract (chocolate-flavored)

1 tsp dark chocolate chips

Directions:

Take a blender and add dark chocolate (or whey protein), stevia, heavy whipping cream (or coconut milk), ice, stevia, chia seeds, water, and cacao.

Now add the extra virgin coconut oil or MCT oil and blend on high until the contents are smooth.

Transfer to a glass and top it with dark chocolate chips.

Serve with ice cubes.

Nutrition: Calories: 570; Fat: 46 g; Carbohydrate: 4.4 g; Protein: 25 g

3 Green Smoothie

Preparation Time: 10 minutes

Cooking Time: 0 minutes

Servings: 6

Ingredients:

1 cup peeled and sliced raw cucumber

1/2 cup peeled and chopped kiwi fruit

1/3 cup fresh pineapple (chopped)

1/2 Hass avocado (scoop the flesh out of the shell after removing the pit)

4 cups water

2 tbsp fresh parsley

1 cup romaine lettuce

1 tbsp maple syrup

1 tbsp chopped fresh ginger (peeled)

Directions:

Put all the ingredients in a blender. Blend on high until smooth. Transfer to a glass and serve with ice cubes.

Nutrition: Calories: 37; Fat: 3 g; Carbohydrate: 2 g; Protein: 1 g

4 Avocado, Chia Seeds & Cacao Smoothie

Preparation Time: 15 minutes

Cooking Time: 0 minutes

Servings: 2

Ingredients:

½ frozen avocado

1 tbsp chia seeds (soak them in 3 tsp water for 10 minutes)

1¼ cups full-fat coconut milk

1 tbsp coconut oil

2 tsp cacao nibs or cocoa powder

¼ cup water (if required)

1 tbsp almond butter (or any nut butter of your choice)

Cacao nibs and cinnamon (for toppings)

Ice (1 small scoop)

Directions:

Add all the ingredients to a high-powered blender. Blend on high until it combines well. Add water if the consistency is too thick.

Transfer to a glass and top it with cinnamon and cacao nibs. Serve with ice (you can avoid the ice if you are not comfortable).

Nutrition: Calories: 394.5; Fat: 40.1 g; Carbohydrate: 11.64 g; Protein: 3.68 g

5 Summer Blackcurrant Smoothie

Preparation Time: 15 minutes

Cooking Time: 0 minutes

Servings: 2

Ingredients:

¼ cup fresh/frozen strawberries (around 3 strawberries)

¼ cup coconut milk OR 4 tbsp heavy whipping cream

½ cup fresh/frozen blackcurrants

2 tbsp powdered/whole chia seeds

½ cup water

½ vanilla bean or ½ tsp vanilla extract (sugar-free)

5-7 drops liquid Stevia extract (optional)

Directions:

Add all the ingredients into a high-powered blender. Blend on high until it combines well. Add water to get a smoothie consistency (not too thick). Let it sit for 5 minutes. Transfer to a glass and serve cold.

Nutrition: Calories: 228; Fat: 17.3 g; Carbohydrate: 8.7 g; Protein: 5.1 g

6 Raspberry Avocado Smoothie

Preparation Time: 10 minutes

Cooking Time: 0 minutes

Servings: 2

Ingredients:

½ cup frozen raspberries (unsweetened) or other low carb frozen berries

1 1/3 cup water

1 ripe avocado (peel and remove the pit)

1 tsp maple syrup (or sugar equivalent)

3 tbsp lemon juice

Directions:

Add all the ingredients into a high-powered blender. Blend on high until it combines well. Add water to get not-so-thick consistency (should be smooth). Transfer to a glass and serve cold.

Nutrition: Total Calories: 227; Fat: 20 g; Carbohydrate: 10.8 g; Protein: 2.5 g

7 Coconut Chia Blueberry Smoothies

Preparation Time: 10 minutes

Cooking Time: 0 minutes

Servings: 4

Ingredients:

1 cup blueberries (frozen)

½ cup coconut cream (take the thick creamy stuff from the top of the can of full-fat coconut milk)

1 cup full-fat coconut milk yogurt

1 cup cashew/almond milk (unsweetened)

2 tbsp powdered chia seeds

2 tbsp sugar-free maple syrup

2 tbsp coconut oil

Directions:

Add all the ingredients to a high-powered blender. Blend on high until it combines well. Add a little almond milk if the consistency is too thick. Transfer to a glass and serve cold.

Nutrition: Total Calories: 249; Fat: 21.07 g; Carbohydrate: 11.26 g; Protein: 6.23 g

8 Vanilla Keto Smoothie

Preparation Time: 10 minutes

Cooking Time: 0 minutes

Servings: 1

Ingredients:

¼ cup vanilla/plain whey protein

2 tbsp chia seeds OR 2 tbsp coconut or almond butter

½ cup full-fat coconut milk OR soured cream

¼ cup water + ½ cup ice

1 vanilla bean OR 1 tsp vanilla extract

1 tbsp extra virgin coconut oil or MCT oil

3-5 drops Stevia extract

Directions:

Take a high-powered blender and place the vanilla or whey protein, water, ice, stevia, and full-fat coconut milk (or sour cream) into it.

Blend until smooth.

Now add the coconut butter or chia seeds and the MCT oil (or extra virgin coconut oil) to the blender.

Blend again until you get a smooth consistency.

Add water if it is too thick.

Transfer to a glass and serve with ice.

Nutrition: Calories: 566; Fat: 45.2 g; Carbohydrate: 5.1 g; Protein: 34.6 g

9 Coconut Mocha Frappe

Preparation Time: 10 minutes

Cooking Time: 0 minutes

Servings: 2

Ingredients:

2 cups high-fat coconut milk (unsweetened)

½ tsp cocoa powder (unsweetened)

1 packet stevia (3.5 oz)

2 tsp instant coffee

Coconut extract (1 drop)

Dark chocolate chips (toppings)

Directions:

Take a large cup and add all the ingredients to it.

Stir well until combined thoroughly (in case it doesn't incorporate well, not to worry!)

Take a shallow freezer-safe bowl. Place this cup into the bowl and freeze it.

Keep scraping the mixture with the fork every couple of hours

Leave it on the counter after the contents have completely frozen. This will soften it up a bit.

Now, transfer it to a high-powered blender and process.

Transfer the frappe to a glass and top it with chocolate chips.

Serve chilled.

Nutrition: Calories: 120; Fat: 10 g; Carbohydrate: 2 g; Protein: 0 g

10   Minty Green Smoothie

Preparation Time: 15 minutes

Cooking Time: 0 minutes

Servings: 1

Ingredients:

1 cup spinach (fresh)

6-8 drops Liquid Stevia Peppermint Sweet Drops

½ avocado (scoop the flesh)

½ cup almond milk (unsweetened)

¼ tsp peppermint extract

1 tsp whey protein powder

1 cup ice

Directions:

Add spinach, protein powder, avocado, and almond milk into a high-powered blender

Blend on high until it combines well

Add Liquid Stevia Peppermint Sweet Drops, ice, and the peppermint extract and blend again.

The smoothie needs to be thick. Add more stevia if you need it sweet.

Transfer to a glass and serve cold.

Nutrition: Calories: 282; Fat: 20 g; Carbohydrate: 9 g; Protein: 10 g

Desserts Recipes

1 Slice-and-Bake Vanilla Wafers

Preparation Time: 10 minutes

Cooking Time: 15 minutes

Servings: 2

Ingredients:

175 g (1¾ cups) blanched almond flour

½ cup granulated erythritol-based sweetener

1 stick (½ cup) unsalted softened butter

2 tbsp Coconut flour

¼ tsp salt

½ tsp vanilla extract

Directions:

Beat the sweetener and butter using an electric mixer in a large bowl for 2 minutes until it becomes fluffy and light. Then beat in the salt, vanilla extract, coconut flour, and almond until thoroughly mixed.

Evenly spread the dough between two sheets of parchment or wax paper and wrap each portion into a size with a diameter of about 1½ inches. Then wrap in paper and refrigerate for 1-2 hours.

Heat the oven to 325°F and line a baking sheet using silicone baking mats or parchment paper. Slice the dough into ¼-inch slices using a sharp knife. Put the sliced dough on the baking sheets and make sure to leave a 1-inch space between wafers.

Place in the oven for about 5 minutes. Slightly flatten the cookies using a flat-bottomed glass. Bake for another 8-10 minutes.

Nutrition: Protein: 2.2 g; Fat: 9.3 g; Carbs: 2.5 g; Erythritol: 6 g; Fiber: 1.3 g; Calories: 101

2 Amaretti

Preparation Time: 15 minutes

Cooking Time: 22 minutes

Servings: 2

Ingredients:

½ cup of granulated erythritol-based sweetener

165 g (2 cups) sliced almonds

¼ cup of powdered of erythritol-based sweetener

4 large egg whites

Pinch of salt

½ tsp almond extract

Directions:

Heat the oven to 300°F and use parchment paper to line two baking sheets. Grease the parchment slightly.

Process the powdered sweetener, granulated sweetener, and sliced almonds in a food processor until it appears like coarse crumbs.

Beat the egg whites plus the salt and almond extract using an electric mixer in a large bowl until they hold soft peaks. Fold in the almond mixture so that it becomes well combined.

Drop a spoonful of the dough onto the prepared baking sheet and allow for a space of one inch between them. Press a sliced almond into the top of each cookie.

Bake in the oven for 22 minutes until the sides become brown. They will appear jelly-like when they are taken out from the oven but will begin to firm as it cools down.

Nutrition: Fat: 8.8 g; Carbs: 4.1 g; Protein: 5.3 g; Fiber: 2.3 g; Erythritol: 18 g; Calories: 117

3 Peanut Butter Cookies for Two

Preparation Time: 5 minutes

Cooking Time: 12 minutes

Servings: 1

Ingredients:

1½ tbsp creamy salted peanut butter

1 tbsp unsalted softened butter

2 tsp lightly beaten egg

2 tbsp granulated erythritol-based sweetener

¼ tsp of vanilla extract

2 tbsp of defatted peanut flour

Pinch of salt

2 tsp sugarless chocolate chips

⅛ tsp baking powder

Directions:

Heat the oven to 325°F, and line a baking sheet with a silicone baking mat or parchment paper.

Beat in the sweetener, butter, and peanut butter using an electric mixer in a small bowl until it is thoroughly mixed.

Add the salt, baking powder, and peanut flour and mix until the dough clumps together. Cut the dough into two and shape each of them into a ball.

Position the dough ball into the coated baking sheets and flatten into a circular shape about half an inch thick. Garnish the dough tops with a teaspoon of chocolate chips. Gently press them into the dough to make them stick.

Bake for 10-12 minutes until golden brown.

Nutrition: Fat: 13.2 g; Carbs: 5.7 g; Protein: 4.9 g; Erythritol: 16 g; Fiber: 1.9 g; Calories: 163

4 Cream Cheese Cookies

Preparation Time: 15 minutes

Cooking Time: 12 minutes

Servings: 6

Ingredients:

¼ cup (½ stick) unsalted softened butter

½ cup (4 oz.) softened cream cheese

1 large egg, at room temperature

½ of cup granulated erythritol-based sweetener

150 g (1½ cups) of blanched almond flour

1 tsp baking powder

½ tsp vanilla extract

Powdered erythritol-based sweetener (for dusting)

¼ tsp of salt

Directions:

Heat the oven to 350°F, and line with a silicone baking mat or parchment paper.

Beat the butter and cream cheese using an electric mixer in a large bowl until it appears smooth. Add the sweetener and keep beating. Beat in the vanilla extract and the egg.

Whisk in the salt, baking powder, and almond flour in a medium bowl. Add the flour mixture into the cream cheese and until well incorporated.

Drop spoonfuls of the dough onto the coated baking sheet. Flatten the cookies.

Bake for 10-12 minutes. Dust with powdered sweetener when cool.

Nutrition: Fat: 13.7 g; Carbs: 3.4 g; Protein: 4.1 g; Erythritol: 10 g; Fiber: 1.5 g; Calories: 154

5 Mocha Cream Pie

Preparation Time: 15 minutes

Cooking Time: 5 minutes

Servings: 10

Ingredients:

1 cup strongly brewed coffee, at room temperature

1 easy chocolate pie crust

1 cup heavy whipping cream

1½ tsp grass-fed gelatin

1 tsp vanilla extract

¼ cup cocoa powder

½ cup powdered erythritol-based sweetener

Directions:

Grease a 9-inch glass or ceramic pie pan. Press the crust mixture evenly and firmly to the sides of the greased pan or its bottom. Refrigerate until the filling is prepared.

Pour the coffee into a small saucepan and add gelatin. Whisk thoroughly and then place over medium heat. Allow it to simmer, whisking from time to time to make sure the gelatin dissolves. Allow it to cool for 20 minutes.

Add the vanilla extract, cocoa powder, sweetener, and the cream into a large bowl. Use an electric mixer to beat until it holds stiff peaks.

Add gelatin mixture that has been cooled and beat until it is well incorporated. Pour over the cooled crust and place in the refrigerator for 3 hours until it becomes firm.

Nutrition: Fat: 20.2 g; Carbs: 6.2 g; Protein: 4.7 g; Erythritol: 18 g; Fiber: 3.1 g; Calories: 218

6 Coconut Custard Pie

Preparation Time: 10 minutes

Cooking Time: 50 minutes

Servings: 8

Ingredients:

1 cup heavy whipping cream

¾ cup powdered erythritol-based sweetener

½ cup full-fat coconut milk

4 large eggs

½ stick (¼ cup) of cooled, unsalted, melted butter

1¼ cups unsweetened shredded coconut

3 tbsp coconut flour

½ tsp baking powder

½ tsp vanilla extract

¼ tsp salt

Directions:

Heat the oven to 350°F and grease a 9-inch ceramic pie pan or glass.

Place the melted butter, eggs, coconut milk, sweetener, and cream in a blender. Blend well.

Add the vanilla extract, baking powder, salt, coconut flour, and a cup of shredded coconut. Continue blending.

Empty the mixture into the pie pan and sprinkle with the rest of the shredded coconut. Bake for 40-50 minutes. Stop when the center is jiggly but the sides are set.

Take out of the oven and allow it to cool for 30 minutes. Place in the refrigerator and allow to stay for 2 hours before cutting it.

Nutrition: Fat: 29.5 g; Carbs: 6.7 g; Protein: 5.3 g; Erythritol: 22.5 g; Fiber: 2.6 g; Calories: 317

7 Dairy-Free Fruit Tarts

Preparation Time: 15 minutes

Cooking Time: 15 minutes

Servings: 2

Ingredients:

1 cup coconut whipped cream

½ easy shortbread crust (dairy-free option)

Fresh mint sprigs

½ cup mixed fresh berries

Directions:

Grease two 4-inch pans with detachable bottoms. Pour the shortbread mixture into pans and firmly press into the edges and bottom of each pan. Refrigerate for 15 minutes.

Loosen the crust carefully to remove from the pan.

Distribute the whipped cream between the tarts and evenly spread to the sides. Refrigerate for 1-2 hours to make it firm.

Use the berries and sprig of mint to garnish each of the tarts.

Nutrition: Fat: 28.9 g; Carbs: 8.3 g; Protein: 5.8 g; Erythritol: 22.5 g; Fiber: 3 g; Calories: 306

8 Strawberry Rhubarb Crisp

Preparation Time: 10 minutes

Cooking Time: 30 minutes

Servings: 2

Ingredients:

Topping Ingredients:

1 tbsp unsweetened shredded coconut

2½ tbsp blanched almond flour

1½ tsp finely chopped pecans

1 tbsp of granulated erythritol-based sweetener

Pinch of salt

2 tsp melted, unsalted butter

¼ tsp ground cinnamon

Filling Ingredients:

⅓ cup sliced fresh strawberries

½ cup chopped fresh rhubarb

1/16 tsp of Xanthan gum

1 tbsp granulated erythritol-based sweetener

Directions:

Preparing the Topping Ingredients:

Heat the oven to 300°F and line a baking sheet with parchment paper.

Whisk the cinnamon, pecans, salt, sweetener, coconut, and almond flour in a medium bowl. Add the melted butter into the mixture, and stir until the resulting mixture appears like coarse crumbs.

Place on the coated baking sheet and firmly press down to make it flat.

Preparing the Filling and Assembling Ingredients:

Heat the oven to 400°F.

Add all the filling ingredients in a medium bowl and make sure that you thoroughly mix them. Place into an 8-oz ramekin and cover with foil.

Nutrition: Calories: 135; Fat: 11.5 g; Protein: 2.6 g; Carbs: 6.3 g; Fiber: 2.6 g; Erythritol: 15 g

9 Raspberry Fool

Preparation Time: 15 minutes

Cooking Time: 0 minutes

Servings: 4

Ingredients:

2-4 tbsp of powdered and divided erythritol-based sweetener

1 cup thawed frozen raspberries

Fresh berries, for garnish

1 cup whipped cream

Directions:

Process 2 tablespoons of sweetener and berries in a food processor or blender until smooth.

Fold in the raspberry puree, leaving some streaks.

Pour mixture into four dessert cups.

Garnish with the berries.

Nutrition: Fat: 20.1 g; Carbs: 5.2 g; Protein: 1.7 g; Erythritol: 15 g; Fiber: 1 g; Calories: 226

10. Cannoli Dessert Dip

Preparation Time: 10 minutes

Cooking Time: 0 minutes

Servings: 8

Ingredients:

¾ cup (6 oz.) of softened cream cheese

1 cup whole-milk ricotta cheese, at room temperature

½ tsp vanilla extract

¾ cup powdered erythritol-based sweetener (plus an additional amount for sprinkling)

⅓ cup sugarless chocolate chips

½ cup of heavy whipping cream

Directions:

Blend the vanilla extract, sweetener, cream cheese, and ricotta in a food processor or blender until smooth.

Whisk in the cream using an electric mixer in a medium bowl until it holds solid peaks. Carefully fold in the chocolate chips and the ricotta mixture and save some for later to sprinkle on top.

Nutrition: Fat: 17.9 g; Carbs: 5.6 g; Protein: 5.7 g; Erythritol: 22.5 g; Fiber: 1.3 g; Calories: 219

Condiments and Sauces Recipes

1 Low Carb BBQ Sauce

Preparation Time: 10 minutes

Cooking Time: 5 minutes

Servings: 1 -16 oz

Ingredients:

¼ cup Lakanto Gold dark colored sugar substitute OR sugar of your choice (Use code MELISSA20 at checkout to save!)

¼ cup apple cider vinegar

¼ cup white vinegar

½ cup water

2 tbsp genuine spread

1 would tomato be able to glue

1 tsp garlic powder

1 tsp onion powder

1 tsp dry yellow mustard

1 tsp salt

1 tsp cayenne pepper (discretionary)

1 tsp fluid smoke (discretionary)

Directions:

If you like a thinner sauce, add more water until the desired thickness is achieved.

If you like an increasingly acrid sauce, add more vinegar.

Go simple with the fluid smoke, a little is enough!

This formula is effectively versatile to various sugars. Utilizing a white sugar will bring about a sauce that is increasingly red in color.

The margarine makes a pleasant lustrous completion and makes the sauce to be on whatever you brush it on.

Nutrition: Calories: 35; Total Fat: 0.4 g; Cholesterol: 0 mg; Sodium: 1198 mg; Total Carbs: 5.9g; Fiber: 1.4 g; Sugars: 3 g; Protein: 1.3 g

2 Tzatziki

Preparation Time: 10 minutes

Cooking Time: 0 minutes

Servings: 8

Ingredients:

½ cup shredded cucumber, drained

1 tsp salt

1 tbsp olive oil

1 tbsp fresh mint, finely chopped

2 garlic cloves

1 cup full-fat Greek yogurt

1 tsp lemon juice

Directions:

Place shredded cucumber in a strainer for an hour or squeeze out moisture through a cheesecloth. Mix all ingredients in a medium bowl. Refrigerate. Use as a vegetable dip, a dip for dehydrated vegetables, or as a sauce for lamb, beef, or chicken. It is also a perfect accompaniment for fried summer squash.

Nutrition: Calories: 79; Carbohydrates: 3 g; Protein: 1 g; Fat: 7 g

3   Satay Sauce

Preparation Time: 10 minutes

Cooking Time: 15 minutes

Servings: 4

Ingredients:

1 can (14 oz) coconut cream (if you can't find coconut cream, coconut milk works well)

1 dry red pepper, seeds removed, chopped fine

1 clove garlic, minced

¼ cup gluten-free soy sauce

⅓ cup natural unsweetened peanut butter

Salt and pepper

Directions:

Place all ingredients in a small saucepan. Bring the mixture to a boil.

Stir while heating to mix peanut butter with other ingredients as it melts.

After the mixture boils, turn down the heat to simmer on low heat for 5 to 10 minutes.

Remove from heat when the sauce is at the desired consistency. Adjust seasoning to taste.

This is a good sauce for chicken or turkey. Just add the sauce during the last minutes of baking or grilling. It can also be used as a dipping sauce.

Nutrition: Calories: 312; Carbohydrates: 7 g; Protein: 7 g; Fat: 30 g

4 Thousand Island Salad Dressing

Preparation Time: 5 minutes

Cooking Time: 5 minutes

Servings: 8

Ingredients:

2 tbsp olive oil

¼ cup frozen spinach, thawed

2 tbsp dried parsley

1 tbsp dried dill

1 tsp onion powder

½ tsp salt

¼ tsp black pepper

1 cup full-fat mayonnaise

¼ cup full-fat sour cream

Directions:

Combine all ingredients in a small mixing bowl. Chill.

Nutrition: Calories: 312; Carbohydrates: 2 g; Protein: 1 g; Fat: 34 g

5 Hollandaise Sauce

Preparation Time: 10 minutes

Cooking Time: 15 minutes

Servings: 4

Ingredients:

4 egg yolks

2 tbsp lemon juice

1½ sticks of butter, melted

Salt and pepper

Directions:

Heat water to boil in a saucepan.

Separate the eggs. Save the whites for another use.

Place the yolks in a heat-resistant bowl, either glass or stainless steel.

Carefully melt the butter in a saucepan without burning.

Place the bowl with the egg yolks over the simmering water to gently heat the eggs. Make sure the water is not touching the bottom of the bowl. The eggs need to be steamed, not cooked.

Add lemon juice to egg yolks.

Slowly stream the melted butter into the egg yolks while whisking. Start with a few drops of butter and then add a slow stream. Whisk the eggs the entire time until all the butter has been added and the sauce has thickened.

Season to taste with lemon juice, salt, and pepper. You can also add a dash of Tabasco sauce.

Serve over poached eggs or cooked vegetables.

Nutrition: Calories: 566; Carbohydrates: 1 g; Protein: 3 g; Fat: 62 g

6 Lemon and Dill Butter

Preparation Time: 15 minutes

Cooking Time: 0 minutes

Servings: 2-3

Ingredients:

2 tbsp cream cheese

5 oz. butter

¼ bunch of dill leaves (approx. 1 oz.)

1 large lemon

½ tsp sea salt

¼ tsp ground black pepper

Directions:

Wash the dill leaves properly under some running water. Ensure that all the dirt is removed and then place them on a cutting board. Using a sharp knife, finely chop the dill leaves and set aside.

Heat a small pan over low heat and melt some butter in it. Once done, allow it to come to room temperature.

Slice up the lemon into two halves and squeeze out as much juice as you can.

In a bowl, combine the butter with some cream cheese, lemon juice, salt, ground pepper and mix well using a spoon.

Add chopped dill and mix again. You can also use a hand blender to whisk all the ingredients together. Store in an airtight container for 2-3 days in the refrigerator until further use.

Nutrition: Calories: 294; Fat: 33 g; Carbohydrate: 1 g; Protein: 1 g

7 Spicy Keto Pimiento Cheese

Preparation Time: 15 minutes

Cooking Time: 0 minutes

Servings: 2-3

Ingredients:

5 tbsp mayonnaise

4 tbsp pickled jalapenos

1 tsp smoked paprika

1 tbsp Dijon mustard

1-inch cayenne pepper

4 oz. cheddar cheese

Some chopped parsley

Directions:

Add mayonnaise to a bowl and whisk using a spoon until it's nice and fluffy. You can also use a hand blender to whisk the mixture.

Place the jalapenos on a cutting board and chop it up roughly using a sharp kitchen knife. Add them to the whisked mayonnaise.

Now slide in some chopped parsley, cheddar cheese, cayenne pepper, and Dijon mustard and whisk again.

Store in an airtight container for 2-3 days in the refrigerator until further use.

Nutrition: Calories: 246; Fat: 24; Carbohydrate: 1 g; Protein: 7 g

8 Keto Chimichurri

Preparation Time: 20 minutes

Cooking Time: 0 minutes

Servings: 6

Ingredients:

1 large lemon

1 small yellow or green bell pepper

1 green chili pepper

1 cup olive oil

A handful of fresh parsley

2 pressed garlic cloves

¼ tsp salt

1/8 tsp ground black pepper

Directions:

Slice the lemon into two halves, and squeeze out as much juice as you can and grate the zest. Make sure you only use the yellow part of the lemon peel and not the white layer.

Wash the bell pepper thoroughly under running water and pat it dry using paper towels. Slice it up and remove its seeds. Using a sharp knife, finely chop the bell pepper along with the green chili and add it to a food processor.

Clean the parsley leaves and place them on a cutting board. Chop them up roughly using a kitchen knife and add them to the food processor along with garlic cloves, salt, pepper, olive oil, and chili pepper and whisk as per the desired consistency.

Store the chimichurri in an airtight container for up to 7 days in the refrigerator until further use.

Nutrition: Calories: 328; Fat: 36 g; Carbohydrate: 0.5 g; Protein: 4 g

9 Keto Chili Aioli

Preparation Time: 18 minutes

Cooking Time: 0 minutes

Servings: 4

Ingredients:

1 large egg

2 garlic cloves

¾ cup avocado oil

½ tsp red chili flakes

½ tsp salt

¼ tsp ground black pepper

1 tbsp lemon juice

3 tbsp Greek yogurt

Directions:

Crack the egg and separate the yolk from the white. Add the yolk to a bowl and whisk well using a spoon. You can also use a hand blender to whisk it slightly. Just remember not to turn it fluffy.

Add the oil slowly to the bowl while stirring it continuously with a spoon or a whisker.

Now add the yogurt along with chili flakes, salt, pepper, Greek yogurt, lemon juice, garlic cloves, and avocado oil and whisk once again using a hand blender.

Add some more salt or lemon as per your desire, and store in an airtight container for up to 2 days in the refrigerator until further use.

Nutrition: Calories: 413; Fat: 46 g; Carbohydrate: 1 g; Protein: 1 g

10   Chipotle Mayonnaise

Preparation Time: 20 minutes

Cooking Time: 0 minutes

Servings: 4

Ingredients:

1 cup mayonnaise

½ tbsp chipotle powder

1 tbsp thick tomato paste

¼ tsp sea salt

Directions:

In a bowl, add the mayonnaise along with the tomato paste, sea salt, and chipotle powder and mix well using a spoon. You can also use some more chipotle powder if you like this dip to be even spicier.

Note: The tomato paste is added predominantly for giving this dip a nice color. You can achieve the same by adding a bit of more chipotle powder.

Let this mixture sit in the refrigerator for at least 30 minutes before you are ready to use it. It might take a day for the flavors to develop.

Store the mayonnaise in an airtight container for up to 7 days in the refrigerator until further use.

Nutrition: Calories: 387; Fat: 42 g; Carbohydrate: 1 g; Protein: 1 g

Chapter 5. The 21-Day Meal Plan

Day	Breakfast	Lunch	Snacks	Dinner
Day 1	French Omelet	Melt-in-Your-Mouth Ribs	Baked Carrot with Bacon	Artichoke and Avocado Pasta Salad
Day 2	Sage Sausage Party	Mom's Meatballs in Creamy Sauce	Standard Greek Salad	Simple Tuna Salad
Day 3	Feta Frittata	Oven-baked Brie Cheese	Creamy Mushroom with Garlic and Thyme	Creamy Chicken Salad
Day 4	Ham Steak with Baco, Mushrooms, and Gruyere	Mexican-Style Pork Chops	Easy Roasted Broccoli	Broccoli Quinoa Casserole
Day 5	Mushroom-Mascarpone Frittata	Easy Pork Tenderloin Gumbo	Roasted Cabbage with Bacon	Apple Arugula and Turkey Salad in a Jar
Day 6	Broccoli Quiche Cups	Pork and Carrot Mini Muffins	Baked Radish Snack	Summertime Slaw
Day 7	Savory Chicken Sausage-Apple	Bacon Blue Cheese Fat Bombs	Boiled Asparagus with Sliced Lemon	Zucchini and Tomato Spaghetti

Day 8	Manchego and Shitake Scramble	Creole-Style Pork Shank	Stuffed Eggs with Bacon-Avocado Flour	White Bean Salad
Day 9	Three-Cheese Quiche	German Pork Rouladen	Spicy Zucchini Chips	Lentil Bolognese
Day 10	Breakfast Turkey Sausage	Rich Pork and Bacon Meatloaf	Cucumber Salad with Tomatoes and Feta	Kale, Lemon, and White Bean Soup
Day 11	No-Bread Breakfast Sandwich	Pork and Vegetable Souvlaki	Quesadillas – Keto Style	Espetada
Day 12	Baked Eggs	Pork Cutlets with Kale	Cheeseburger Tomatoes	Chicken Caprese Salad with Avocado
Day 13	Cured Salmon with Chives and Scrambled Eggs	Italian Keto Plate	Strawberry Avocado Smoothie	Creamy Chicken with Salami and Olives
Day 14	Eggs Benedict on Avocados	Steak Tartare	Chocolate Keto Smoothie	Buffalo Wings, Hot Sauce & Blue Cheese Dip
Day 15	Keto Chaffles	Keto Deviled Eggs	Green Smoothie	Chicken Francese
Day 16	Keto Taco Cups	Garlic Butter Salmon with	Avocado, Chia Seeds & Cacao	Tacos

		Lemon Asparagus Skillet	Smoothie	
Day 17	Loaded Cauliflower Salad	Hearty Shrimp Curry	Summer Blackcurrant Smoothie	Chicken Livers
Day 18	Caprese Zoodles	Ancient Salmon Glaze and Teriyaki	Raspberry Avocado Smoothie	Garlic Chicken Low-Card
Day 19	Keto Broccoli and Cheddar Soup	Extremely Low Carb Chicken and Pepper Soup	Coconut Chia Blueberry Smoothie	Keto Buffalo Drumsticks With Chili Aioli And Garlic
Day 20	Egg Roll Bowls	Butter Fried Kale and Pork with Cranberries	Vanilla Keto Smoothie	Chicken and Herb Butter with Keto Zucchini Roll-ups
Day 21	Three Cheese Chicken and Cauliflower		Coconut Mocha Frappe	Keto Buffalo Drumsticks With Chili Aioli and Garlic

Chapter 6. Forbidden Food list

You should be minimizing the following categories of food when you are trying to implement the keto diet.

Starch and Carbs

Avoid starch and excess intake of carbohydrates as much as you can. This means that you will have to get rid of most of your staple dishes such as porridge, pasta, rice, mashed potatoes, and bread. I know this can be quite difficult to implement in the beginning. Recent research has found that refined carbohydrates predict insulin resistance, which will cause inflammation and other related cardiovascular disorders.

I love carbs so this was the hardest for me to avoid. However you will soon realize that the benefits of keeping them off your plate are several and that should motivate you to avoid them.

Sugar (and Potential Sweetener Alternatives)

It goes without saying here that elimination of sugar-rich food is a must when you are following the keto diet or any other diet. Sugar causes inflammation in your body. Excessively sweet desserts should be avoided at all costs.

You can maybe sneak in a tiny piece of homemade cake or dessert every now and then to satisfy that sweet tooth until you adopt the keto diet completely! This is extremely hard for many to do but I understand it. I treat myself to one or two pieces of dark chocolate with at least 70% cacao or higher with my evening cup of coffee.

If you just can't do without the taste of sugar or the sweetness associated with it either added to your beverages or to food, there are a few options I would recommend.

However, if you can do without any sweeteners, this will be your best choice especially if you are doing intermittent fasting with the keto diet. The taste of a sweetener whether it has calories or not will break your fast.

There are sweeteners derived from natural sources which undergo varying amounts of processing.

- Erythritol:
    - Erythritol is a natural, almost calorie-free, and zero net-carb sweetener that is a sugar alcohol. It has approximately 60% to 80% of the sweetness of sugar. It is derived from fruits and tastes like cane sugar.
    - Erythritol is created by fermenting the natural sugars found in a variety of fruits.
        - However, erythritol products available to consumers are usually derived from corn so it is important to find non-GMO products if you are concerned about consuming genetically modified products.
        - These products are available in granulated and very fine powdered form so that erythritol can be used for baking and be easily included in other food products.
    - While it has been determined that erythritol does not cause any serious side effects, be aware that some may experience some digestive issues. Please refer to published research.
- Monk Fruit:
    - Monk fruit originated from the southern mountains of China. It is sometimes referenced by the name *lo han guo*. It is said that the name came from Buddhist monks who first discovered and cultivated it sometime around the 13th century.
    - Monk fruit is a zero-calorie natural sweetener that is 300-400 times sweeter than cane sugar.

- - It has powerful antioxidants called mogrosides which are used by our body differently than natural sugars. Please refer to research.
    - It also has anti-inflammatory properties. Please refer to research.
    - It is used to help reduce the risk of obesity and diabetes. Please refer to research.
  - Monk fruit sweeteners are created by removing the seeds and skin, crushing the fruit, and obtaining the juice. The no-calorie juice is used in food and beverages to reduce your sugar intake without losing the sweetness of sugar.
  - To create a granulated form of monk fruit, it is dried and ground into a powder form and may be combined with other sweeteners. You may not find it available for purchase in retail stores, but it is now commonly used in the U.S. by many consumer packaged and beverage companies in numerous food products including yogurt, fruit bowl, bakery items, ice creams, coffee drinks, soft drinks. It continues to grow in popularity.

- Stevia:
  - Stevia is about 50-350 times sweeter than sugar.
  - Thus far, recent stevia studies have been promising about its potential benefits against atherosclerosis glucose control, carcinogenesis, and hypertension, and inflammation.
  - Be aware that the unprocessed version of stevia does have a strong aftertaste resulting in stevia products that are highly processed and which are often combined with erythritol and other sweeteners. It is important to read the product label for the list of ingredients when making a purchase. You may find out that the stevia product you just purchased has very little stevia in it after all.

Alcohol

Consuming a glass of wine or whiskey occasionally won't do much harm, but make sure that you stay away from beer. Beer is extremely rich in carbs and you should definitely keep that out of the way!

Did you know that hard liquor such as whiskey, vodka, etc. have no carbs as long as you don't add sweet mixers to the alcohol? This doesn't mean you should drink hard liquor excessively as they still have calories. A moderate drink here or there is fine. I love my single malt scotch!

Important Tip to Consider Before Getting Started: Apple Cider Vinegar

You may have heard about utilizing apple cider vinegar as part of your daily keto diet plan. If not, let me explain some of the key benefits of drinking apple cider vinegar and how it will support your keto diet overall health benefits and weight loss.

The acetic acid is sour and has a strong smell that does not taste very good, and I can attest to this. There are ways to reduce the pungent taste by diluting it with 8 ounces of water and adding lemon juice, for example.

Key Health Benefits

One word of caution before I let you know some of the key benefits. If you decide to incorporate apple cider vinegar into your daily routine, I don't recommend that you ever consume apple cider vinegar or other vinegars without diluting it with water due to its acetic acid content. If you don't, the apple cider vinegar may damage or burn your esophagus and possibly damage your tooth enamel.

According to several research studies, it summarized the following points:

- There is evidence that links the use of vinegar to a reduced risk for hypertension (high blood pressure) and cancer.

- There is some evidence that the consumption of vinegar increases short-term fullness or satiety which reduces your appetite.

There is some animal research that documents the ability of apple cider vinegar or vinegar to assist with fat loss to complement the keto diet. Some of the ways to support fat loss include the following:

- Reduction in obesity – Results indicate that acetic acid has effects on the lipid metabolism in the liver and the skeletal muscles and thus works against obesity.

- Reduction in body fat accumulation – Results indicate that acetic acid reduces the accumulation of body fat and liver lipids.

- Ability to suppress appetite – The results indicate that acetic acid has a central role in regulating appetite.

As you have been shown through research, there are a number of health benefits by incorporating apple cider vinegar into your daily regimen whether you are on the keto diet or not.

So how do you take advantage of apple cider vinegar? I would suggest you search on YouTube or Google about apple cider vinegar. You will find a lot of information. There will be varying ideas of how to incorporate apple cider vinegar into your diet either by drinking it, adding it to foods, salad dressings, or sauces.

Here is what I do. I drink Certified Bragg Organic Raw Apple Cider Vinegar that is non-GMO, unfiltered, unheated, unpasteurized, and it has 5% acidity.

However, I do not drink it without diluting it first.

- Put 8 oz. of cold water into a glass
- Add 2 tsp of apple cider vinegar
- Add 1 tsp of lemon juice

- If you wish you can add a tsp of pure cranberry juice (nothing added, especially no sugar).

- Mix it well. Keep additional water available to drink after you finished the apple cider vinegar drink to rinse away any residual acetic acid.

Chapter 7. Keto Shopping List for Seniors

Keto Ingredients

Starting out with the very basics, having knowledge about keto-friendly ingredients is going to get you off to a good start. When you need a reminder, just think about fats and dairy. This is the basis of the diet. The following list is an example of some of the top foods that you should be reaching for while following keto:

- Seafood (clams, mussels, oysters, squid, and octopus)
- Low-Carb Vegetables (cauliflower, broccoli, and kale, leafy greens, celery, etc.)
- Cheese (especially organic, grass-fed for healthy levels of Omega-3 fatty acids)
- Avocados
- Meat and Poultry (choose grass-fed beef whenever possible, for healthy Omega-3 fatty acids)
- Eggs (choose varieties with extra Omega-3)
- Coconut Oil (organic, extra virgin)
- Plain Greek Yogurt and Cottage Cheese (choose grass-fed for Omega-3 content)
- Olive Oil (organic, extra virgin)
- Nuts and Seeds (almonds, cashews, sunflower seeds, pecans, macadamia nuts, walnuts, pistachios, pumpkin seeds, and sesame seeds)
- Berries (blueberries, raspberries, blackberries, and strawberries)
- Butter and Cream (again, preference is for grass-fed varieties for Omega-3)
- Olives
- Unsweetened Tea and Coffee

After seeing this list of ingredients, you should be able to visualize how you can put them together in order to create nutritious meals for yourself. You can use this as a basic shopping list for your next trip to the grocery store. Shopping for your new keto diet should not be that much different than your regular shopping trip. You have to be aware of how many carbs are in each ingredient, but otherwise, you have a lot of freedom to decide exactly what you'd like to eat for the week. For this reason, the Keto diet should never become boring or repetitive. You have so many options that you should be able to change up if necessary.

Allow yourself to explore by using keto-friendly ingredients in your meals that you would normally not eat on a regular basis. A handful of flax seeds in your yogurt, for example, can be a nice way to get more of your necessary nutrients without having to change the way that you would normally eat. Being crafty with these additions and substitutions will help you adjust to your new lifestyle. Eating keto does not have to be strict and you will see just how great it will feel to be on a diet that feels like it isn't a diet. Whether you are cooking for yourself or eating outside of your home, you will be able to stick with your diet without too many issues.

At any age, proper nutrition is incredibly important, but as we age, our bodies are going through some major changes. To help with these changes, it will be essential to make certain adjustments to our routines and nutrition. The vital factor to remember is that it is never too late to start taking care of yourself. When you neglect your health after the age of fifty, the effects may become more noticeable than ever before. So, how exactly does age affect our nutritional needs?

Aging and Nutritional Needs

As we age, you can expect a number of different changes to happen in your body, including thinner skin, loss of muscle, and less stomach acid. When these things happen, this can, unfortunately, make you more prone to nutrient deficiencies and overall quality of life. This is where the ketogenic diet comes in handy! By eating a variety of foods and incorporating the proper supplements, you will be able to meet your nutrient needs with no issues! Below, you will find some of the effects of aging and how to help the issue.

Fewer Calories-More Nutrients

On a general basis, an individual's daily calorie count will depend on a number of factors, including activity level, muscle mass, weight, and height. As for us older adults, we will need to begin lowering the number of calories we take in, in order to maintain or lose weight. Generally, older adults tend to exercise and move less compared to younger individuals.

While consuming fewer calories, it is important to continue getting higher levels of nutrients. For this reason, it is highly suggested to consume a variety of foods such as low-carb vegetables and lean meats to help get the proper nutrients and fight against any nutrient deficiencies. The nutrients you will want to focus on including vitamin B12, calcium, and vitamin D, magnesium, potassium, Omega-3 fatty acids, and iron.

Benefits of Fiber

While many people do not like to discuss this, constipation is a prevalent health issue for individuals over the age of 50. In fact, women over the age of 65 are two to three times more likely to experience constipation! This may be due to the fact that people over the age of 50 generally move less and are more likely to be taking a medication that has constipation as an unfortunate side effect.

To help relieve constipation, you will want to make sure you are getting enough fiber. When you eat more fiber, it is able to pass through your gut, undigested, and help regulate bowel movements and form stool. As an added benefit, high-fiber diets may also be able to prevent diverticular disease. Diverticular disease is a condition where small pouches build along the wall of the colon and become inflamed.

Focus on Protein

You learned that it is important not to focus on protein, but it will be essential to find a balance in your new diet. As we age, it is very common to lose both strength and muscle. In fact, on average, an adult will lose anywhere between 3-8% of their muscle mass per decade after the age of 30. When we lose muscle mass, it could lead to poor health, fractures, and weakness among an elderly population. By eating more protein, you can help fight sarcopenia and maintain your muscle mass.

Vitamin B12

As mentioned earlier, keeping up with proper nutrients is going to be vital for your health. One of the vitamins you will want to focus on is Vitamin B12. This is a water-soluble vitamin that is in charge of making red blood cells and keeping your brain healthy. Unfortunately, it is estimated that anywhere from 1-30% of individuals over the age of 50 have a lower ability to absorb this vitamin from their diet.

One of the main reasons individuals over the age of 50 have difficulty absorbing vitamin B12 may be due to the fact that they have reduced stomach acid reduction. Vitamin B12 is bound to proteins. In order for your body to use this vitamin, the stomach acid separates it from the protein and becomes absorbed. To benefit your new diet, you will want to consider taking a supplement of vitamin B12 or consuming foods that are fortified with the vitamin.

Vitamin D and Calcium

When it comes to bone health, calcium and vitamin D are going to be very important. While calcium is in charge of maintaining and building healthy bones, it depends on vitamin D to help the body absorb the calcium in the first place! Unfortunately, adults have a harder time absorbing calcium in their diets. This may be due to the fact that the gut absorbs less calcium as we age. However, the main culprit of a reduction in calcium is typically due to a vitamin D deficiency. As you can tell, they work hand in hand!

The reason we may experience a vitamin D deficiency is due to thinning skin. Generally, our body makes vitamin D from the cholesterol in the skin when it is exposed to sunlight. As the skin becomes thinner, it reduces the ability to make vitamin D and, in turn, reduces the ability to get enough calcium. When these two things happen, it increases the risk of fractures and bone loss.

To help counter this aging effect, you will want to make sure you are getting enough vitamin D and calcium in your diet. Some accessible sources will be dairy products, leafy vegetables, and dark greens. As far as Vitamin D goes, you will want to include a variety of fish or even a Vitamin D supplement such as cod liver oil.

Dehydration

Whether on the ketogenic diet or not, staying hydrated is important at any age. In fact, water makes up about 60% of our bodies! Whether you are 20, 30, or 50 years old, the body still continually loses water through urine and sweat. As we age, it makes us more prone to dehydration.

When we become dehydrated, the water detects the thirst through receptors found all throughout the body and the brain. As we age, the receptors become less sensitive, making it hard to distinguish the thirst in the first place. On top of this, our kidneys are there to help converse water, but they also lose function with age.

Unfortunately, the consequences of dehydration are pretty harsh for the older population. When you are dehydrated long-term, this could reduce your ability to absorb medication and could worsen any medical condition. For this reason, it will be vital you keep up with your intake of water. I suggest trying a water challenge with friends and family or try having a glass of water with each meal you have.

Appetite

One of the last topics we will tackle the subject of aging is the decrease in appetite. While this may seem like a benefit, a lack of eating could lead to a number of different nutritional deficiencies and unwanted weight loss. Poor appetite is most commonly linked to a heightened risk of death and overall poor health.

It is believed that some of the significant factors behind appetite loss could be due to changes in smell, taste, and hormones. Generally, older adults who have lower levels of hunger have higher levels of fullness hormones. When this happens, it causes individuals to be less hungry overall. As we age, the changes in smell and taste can also make food seem less appealing.

If you find this happens to you, you may want to establish a healthy habit of snacking. When you snack, try to reach for keto-friendly foods such as eggs, yogurt, and almonds to help put the nutrients back into your diet. If you are aware of this issue, it is something you can get a grasp on before it becomes a real problem.

Conclusion

You've come a long way to get to this page. Now, you know how to make a plan for changing your eating habits; you know how your lifestyle changes will affect you differently as a woman over 50.

You read all our advice on avoiding the common mistakes women make when they are first starting out with the ketogenic diet. We even went over special exercises that women say help them in their health goals.

Now, your job is to take it from theory to practice. You know all you need to know—only you can make the necessary changes for yourself.

I suspect that the section you will get the most use out of is the 30-day meal plan for keto. Don't feel like you can't stray away from these recipes, however. There are, in fact, other meals outside of this list that still accord to the requirements of the keto diet. You can simply use the recipes on this list to come up with meals of your own, and make modifications as you see fit.

The biggest problem that women have after getting invested in keto is continuing to follow through with their plans. They get inspired to get into it and even do everything right for weeks or even months.

But then something inevitably happens in their life that makes keto a lower priority. The key to prevent this from happening to you is keeping a Keto journal.

In your keto journal, you will keep yourself accountable for your diet and exercise goals. All of them go together to get the results you are looking for: the foods you eat every day and the amount of time you spend in the gym are both things you should write down in your keto journal.

Many women will be very hesitant to do this. Mainly, they are concerned that they will start the journal only to end up leaving it behind. But the first few weeks is when the keto journal matters the most.

You should try to keep up with it as long as you can. Even if you end up leaving it behind later, the keto journal will be a great help to commit yourself to keto. After all, you have your commitments to the lifestyle written on paper.

My final note to you is to be forgiving of yourself. No one—not a single soul—starts the keto lifestyle and sticks with it without making any mistakes. It is no different from any other change that people make to their lives, in this sense.

People who quit smoking for months often find themselves cheating and smoking a cigarette, and they end up picking up cigarettes more and more after that, thinking they have already messed up irredeemably.

This is because we are so used to sticking with our new routine that breaking away from it with our old habits makes it feel like we are getting back to our old selves.

Don't let yourself fall into this trap. Accept right now that you will make a mistake at some point. You will eat a non-keto food; you won't go to the gym on a day you said you would; you won't follow the fasting routine you have set for yourself.

Whatever the goals you set for yourself, you can't be a complete perfectionist about them. Be open to your lifestyle change while also being open to slipping every now and again.

Finally, if you found this book useful in any way, share it with your friends!

CPSIA information can be obtained
at www.ICGtesting.com
Printed in the USA
BVHW091133290421
606134BV00001B/71